UNDERSTANDING CANCER

To the medical, nursing, and support staff
of the Oncology Units in the Mater Hospitals in Dublin,
and in oncology units worldwide,
who combine good humor and skilled dedication
with hope for the future

UNDERSTANDING CANCER

A Scientific and Clinical Guide for the Layperson

by Peter A. Dervan, M.D.

with a foreword by
Christopher D.M. Fletcher, M.D.

McFarland & Company, Inc., Publishers
Jefferson, North Carolina, and London

Library of Congress Cataloguing-in-Publication Data

Dervan, Peter A., 1945–
Understanding cancer : a scientific and clinical guide for the layperson / by Peter A. Dervan; with a foreword by Christopher D.M. Fletcher.
p. cm.
Includes bibliographical references and index.
ISBN 0-7864-0628-3 (sewn softcover : 50# alkaline paper) ∞
1. Cancer—Popular works. I. Title.
RC263.D46 1999
616.99'4—dc21 99-14626
CIP

British Library Cataloguing-in-Publication data are available

Manufactured in the United States of America

McFarland & Company, Inc., Publishers
Box 611, Jefferson, North Carolina 28640
www.mcfarlandpub.com

Contents

List of Illustrations vi

Foreword by Christopher D.M. Fletcher, M.D. 1

Introduction 3

1 • The Scope of the Cancer Problem 5

2 • Cancer through the Ages 11

3 • Tissue Organization and Differentiation 15

4 • The Cell's Response to Stress 23

5 • Precancer, Invasion, and Metastases 30

6 • Common Adult Cancers 39

7 • Childhood Cancers 81

8 • Genes and Cancer 91

9 • What Causes Cancer? 106

10 • How Do Doctors Diagnose Cancer? 121

11 • Treatment Principles and Strategies 131

12 • Where to Get More Information 141

13 • Cancer Screening 145

14 • The Future 159

Appendix: Resources for Cancer Patients and Families 167

Glossary 173

Index 197

List of Illustrations

1.1	New Cancer Cases in the United States	8
1.2	Cancer Deaths in the United States	8
3.1	Normal Cell	16
3.2	Tissue and Organ Differentiation	18
4.1	Benign Nevus (Mole) and Malignant Melanoma	24
4.2	The Cell Cycle and Mitosis	25
4.3	Cell Response to Stress	28
5.1	Clonal Growth of Carcinoma in Situ	31
5.2	Progression of Malignant Changes	32
5.3	Loss of Cell Adhesion	33
6.1	Tumor Differentiation	41
6.2	Microscopic Appearance of Tumor	43
6.3	Lung Cancer	46
6.4	Ductal Carcinoma in Situ (DCIS) of the Breast	52
6.5	Invasive Breast Cancer	53
6.6	Prostate and Bladder Cancer	56
6.7	Cancer of the Esophagus and Stomach	59
6.8	Colorectal Cancer	62
6.9	Leukemia	68
6.10	Multiple Myeloma	70
6.11	Cancer of the Cervix, Uterus, and Ovary	72
6.12	Kidney Cancer	73
8.1	Nuclear Chromatin	92
8.2	DNA Structure	96
8.3	The DNA Encyclopedia	96
8.4	DNA Replication	97

Foreword

Cancer, a term generally used for all types of malignant tumor, is unfortunately very common and accounts for about a quarter of all deaths in the western world. This is especially so because of our increased life expectancy nowadays, since cancer is increasingly common with advancing age. As a consequence, most individuals (and families) come into close contact with cancer patients, be they relatives or friends, at some stage in their lives. People's response to a diagnosis of cancer, rendered for them or for someone else, is remarkably variable. Some people seek all the detailed information, ranging through cause, treatment and likely outcome, that they can, whereas others prefer to entrust everything (including all aspects of decision-making) to their doctors and other carers. The latter response is becoming much less frequent in the modern world of free information and in the face of barrages of (frequently unsolicited!) medical facts and opinions through all forms of the media.

Despite such availability of information there remains enormous ignorance, confusion and hence often heightened fear regarding cancer. This is sometimes made worse by the existence of conflicting data and opinions, some of which reflect the genuinely unresolved nature of certain questions (there are still many problems and uncertainties concerning the development and best treatment of some cancers!) and some of which result from inadequately supported views expressed by fanatics or charlatans.

In the face of this situation, it is, nevertheless, clear that we know more now about cancer than we ever have, that more cancer patients are cured (or live longer) now than ever before and that there is ample evidence that the situation will continue to improve, especially if the promise of new insights from molecular genetics lives up to expectations. Furthermore, while very specialized questions or concerns may arise for individual patients (and, thus, might not be best answered by a broad-based book such as this), nevertheless, there are common and recurring themes which feature repeatedly in the questions asked by cancer patients and those closely associated with them—"Is this type of cancer common?", "Where did it come from?",

"Did something at work or home cause it?", "Is this type of cancer familial?", "Could it have been prevented?", "What tests will be needed?", "What types of treatments are there?", "What are the chances of cure?"

Happily two of the common misconceptions—that cancer is one disease and that there is a cancer "epidemic"—seem gradually to be disappearing. Peter Dervan's marvelous book explains the background to these false impressions and goes much further—it provides clear and very readable information regarding the nature of cancer (in its many forms), where it comes from, how it differs from "normal," how it is diagnosed, how (in general terms) it is treated and what our goals and hopes are for the future. Dr. Dervan also provides more detailed information regarding the commonest types of cancer, such as those in the lung, breast and bowel.

Personally, I believe that Peter has done an absolutely excellent job in rendering a complex subject accessible to a wide relationship—patients, friends and families, other carers and interested lay readers. Ignorance and confusion very often make patients and their loved ones much more afraid than need be—Peter Dervan's book will contribute enormously towards the prevention (or cure) of this problem. I urge anyone who wants to know or understand more about cancer to read this book—there is no doubt in my mind that you will find it helpful.

CHRISTOPHER D.M. FLETCHER, M.D., FRCPath
Professor of Pathology
Harvard Medical School
Boston, Massachusetts

Introduction

No matter what your age, the chances are you know someone who has cancer. The older you are, the more likely you are to know a cancer victim. Possibly, even a friend or relative has died from this disease.

As I entered my forties, it seemed that I knew more and more people with cancer. Friends, relatives, acquaintances seemed to have little or no idea about what exactly cancer is. These included many very well educated people; some had studied biology at college. Judging from the amount of media coverage on television and in magazines, it is obvious that the public is interested in the topic. Yet they have little fundamental understanding about the nature of cancer. Perhaps this is because there are so many different cancers, and medical terminology is confusing. Also, in the past, there was so much taboo associated with cancer that people did not discuss the topic openly.

By the time my forties were ending, cancer had touched my own family, my wife's family, and my neighbors' families. At work, colleagues were affected. The diagnosis of cancer brings a wave of emotional shock and disbelief. Patients become confused, angry, and fearful. One of the biggest psychological problems they face is fear of the unknown. From time to time, friends asked me to recommend some useful books—not too technical and not too spiritual. To my amazement, when I first checked the bookstores, I could find only textbooks and some self-help books on specific cancers. Medical textbooks are not very "user friendly" for the average reader. They are highly technical and full of jargon and assume that the reader already has an understanding of anatomy, cell biology, biochemistry, and physiology. The self-help books often touch superficially on the nature of cancer and do not offer much depth for the reader who really wants to know what exactly is cancer. Because cancer is so common, I am still amazed that bookstores have not filled their shelves with books more like this one.

For some time I had been toying with the idea of writing this book. On my fiftieth birthday, the motivation arrived. What I hope this book will do is give you a good understanding of the essence of cancer. I have tried to bring together the science behind cancer and the clinical aspects of the common cancers. I have attempted to write it in a way that almost anyone can understand. Wherever possible I have substituted plain English for more specific scientific terminology. Simple line drawings illustrate the main ideas in the text.

I hope that readers find *Understanding Cancer* informative and enjoyable, and that it will also remove some of the myth and fear that surrounds this disease. While the book explains the various treatments available for cancer patients, do not expect to find answers to specific medical problems. You can find many self-help textbooks in bookstores, and these often address common problems. Better still, talk to your physician and ask him or her to explain specific problems and treatments.

Although this book is not a self-help book, it contains a full chapter on where to find self-help information. This decade has given us remarkable advances in information technology. It has given us the Internet and the World Wide Web (WWW). The WWW contains an abundance of information for the cancer patient and for all those interested in cancer. I have included many useful WWW addresses.

CHAPTER 1

The Scope of the Cancer Problem

Sixty thousand United States soldiers were killed in the Vietnam war between 1960 and 1975. In 1996 more than 550,000 Americans died from cancer. This disease claims a new victim every minute. Every 12 minutes a woman dies from breast cancer and 4 new patients are given the devastating news that they have this scourge.

We often talk of cancer as if it were a single disease. It is not. It is a group of diseases that have overlapping and often similar characteristics but also have extreme differences. Some cancers grow slowly and are indolent; they require only local removal and have a 100 percent cure rate. Others grow quickly, disseminate widely, resist all forms of therapy, and are invariably fatal. Between these extremes there are dozens of different cancers with a wide spectrum of behavior and responsiveness to treatment.

Just before Christmas in 1971, President Richard M. Nixon declared war on cancer and committed billions of taxpayers' dollars to cancer research. Since 1971 the National Cancer Institute has spent more than $27 billion in its research programs. Many critics publicly castigate this effort as a dismal failure. Ask the thousands of parents whose children have been cured of leukemia during this time. They will not agree. Neither will the surviving victims of prostate or breast cancer. Annual federal funding for research into these cancers would not buy three new fighter planes.

To some extent, however, the critics are correct. Between 1973 and 1992 the overall cancer death rate rose by 6.3 percent. Although we have had amazing insights into the science of cancer during this time, we are still waiting for the cures. The overall cure rates for lung, breast, prostate, intestinal, and ovarian cancers are disappointing. However, researchers have made remarkable breakthroughs in the treatment of childhood cancers, leukemias, lymphomas, and bone and testicular cancers. These cancers are now often curable. In the past they were invariably fatal.

Other little-publicized breakthroughs benefit cancer patients daily.

Surgery is less disfiguring. New limb-sparing surgical techniques spare children from amputations. The dreaded nausea and vomiting associated with chemotherapy is for most patients a thing of the past, due to new highly effective antinausea drugs. Granulocyte stimulating factor, a bioengineered growth factor that stimulates the patient's bone marrow, reduces life-threatening infections. The past twenty-five years have also seen better pain control and the introduction of numerous minor medical devices. These all add up to improved patient care and comfort.

So, if we measure success by our attempts to eradicate the common cancers, then, yes, the efforts of the past twenty-five years have been a failure. However, if we take a broader viewpoint, we can rejoice in many major successes. Furthermore, these new insights are the stepping stones for new victories in our continued war on cancer. Without the accumulated knowledge from the past quarter of a century we would have no chance for future success.

Breast cancer accounts for 20 percent of all female cancer deaths and the public understands its relevance and importance. However, what they do not know is that cancer of the prostate gland kills the same number of men each year. Cancer mortality rates in males and females are similar. Forty percent of Americans get cancer and the risk of dying from cancer is 1 in 4. Figures quoted for the United States (see table 1 and figures 1.1 and 1.2) are similar or identical to statistics available for the rest of the western world. After heart attacks (740,000 deaths annually), cancer is the next biggest killer. These statistics do not apply to Asia or parts of Africa, where the prevalence of different types of cancer is dramatically different. The World Health Organization estimates that cancer kills 6 million people every year.

In the United States, SEER and the National Center for Health Statistics provide comprehensive statistical data. SEER is the Surveillance, Epidemiology, and End Results program of the National Cancer Institute (NCI) in Washington. The NCI is a subdivision of the National Institute of Health. It takes time to collect and analyze data. Normally, there is a delay of one to two years before the results are published. SEER collects data from nine population-based cancer registries in the United States These are located in four metropolitan areas and five states: Atlanta, Georgia (five counties); Detroit, Michigan (three counties); San Francisco–Oakland, California (five counties); Seattle-Puget Sound, Washington (thirteen counties); and all counties in Connecticut, Iowa, Hawaii, New Mexico, and Utah. SEER's recently expanded program includes greater coverage of minority populations, especially Hispanics. It now covers approximately 10 percent of the U.S. population and has information on more than 1.7 million cancer patients. The National Center for Health Statistics collects its mortality statistics from death certificates, and their data account for more than 99 percent of U.S. deaths. Both collecting systems have drawbacks, but for the most part there is an agreement between the two agencies. For white males, SEER data indicate essentially no change in cancer mortality from 1975 to 1988; the National Center for Health Statistics found an increase of about 4 percent.

In 1900 the death rate for cancer per 100,000 population was 63. In 1922 it was 87; in 1991 it was 390. Some readers will find it interesting to note other mortality figures from 1900: tuberculosis was 201, influenza and pneumonia 181, heart disease 123, infant diarrhea and enteritis 108, diabetes mellitus 92, diphtheria 43, typhoid and paratyphoid fevers 39.

In Europe, the European Commission's International Agency for Research on Cancer and the European Network of Cancer Registries keep track of the facts and figures. Most informed observers agree that cancer

Table 1.1. Cancer Statistics, United States (1996)

	New Cases	Deaths
Lung	177,000	158,700
Breast	185,700	44,560
Prostate	317,100	41,400
Pancreas	26,300	27,800
Colorectal	133,500	54,900
Bladder	52,900	11,700
Uterus	49,700	10,900
Ovary	26,700	14,800
Melanoma	38,300	7,300
Kidney	30,600	12,000
Stomach	22,800	14,000
Lymphoma	60,200	24,810
Leukemia	27,600	21,000
All other	210,750	110,870
All sites	**1,359,150**	**554,740**

Table 1 shows the total number of new cases and the deaths from the most important cancers. These figures do not include the commonest of all cancers, namely, squamous and basal cell carcinomas of the skin (about 800,000 new cases each year). These skin cancers are usually cured by excision and rarely can kill and are therefore not included. Malignant melanoma, however, is included. Source: American Cancer Society.

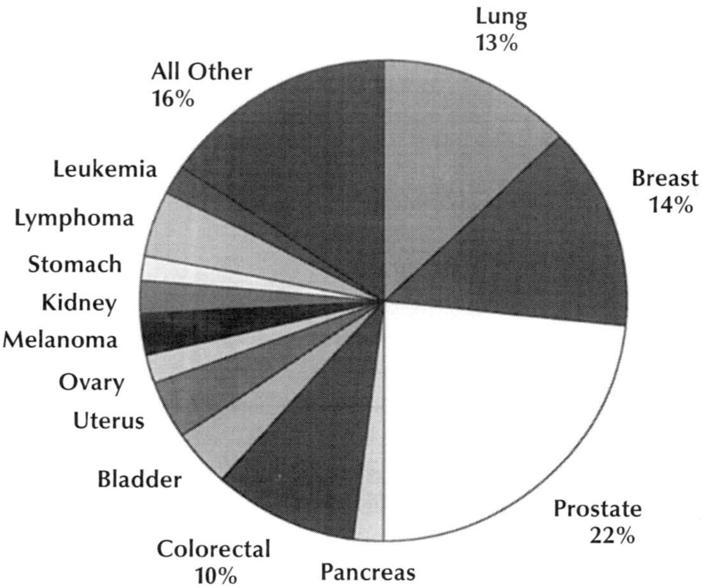

Figure 1.1. Distribution of new cancer cases in the United States in 1996. Source: Data from American Cancer Society.

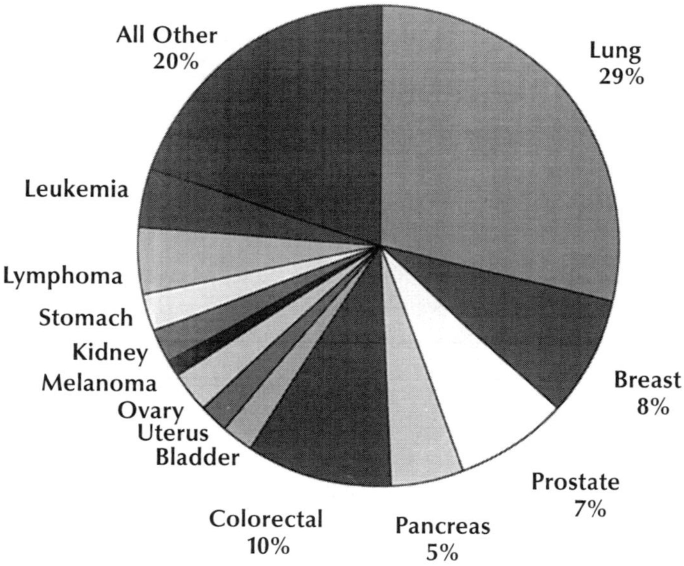

Figure 1.2. Distribution of cancer deaths in the United States in 1996. Source: Data from American Cancer Society.

statistics throughout the western world are similar. However, in a 1991 survey of forty-nine national and international health atlases, consistency in data presentation was poor. If you find somewhat different cancer statistics appearing in different publications and magazines, blame the discrepancy on different methods for collecting and presenting data. Figures 1.1 and 1.2 show the 1996 statistics for new cases and deaths in the United States for the major cancer killers. Not included are 800,000 common skin cancers (other than melanoma), since these rarely kill. Keeping totals on cancer statistics is important. By tracking incidence and mortality trends, epidemiologists get clues about causative agents. Cancer statistics also help them to assess the effects of improved diagnostic, screening, and treatment methods.

Cancer cure is expensive for the individual, the family, and society. The United States spends $104 billion on cancer treatment each year. Loss of work costs $12 billion. Cancer screening—including mammography, pap smears, colorectal examinations, and tests for prostate cancer—costs $4 billion. Moreover, the cost of cancer care, like that of other diseases, is rocketing. High-tech medicine raises the standard of medical care, and the cost. The recent increase in overall incidence is partly due to more accurate reporting and earlier detection of prostate and breast cancer. Since old age is a major risk factor for cancer, much of the increase is explained by the fact that we live longer than our forefathers.

Those who say that we are gradually getting the upper hand in the war on cancer can applaud the fact that, during the past twenty-five years, cancer mortality for men and women under the age of 55 has fallen by 16 percent. More impressively, the overall mortality for children (up to the age of 14), has dropped 42 percent.

Bibliography

Bailar, J.C., and E.M. Smith. Progress against cancer? *New England Journal of Medicine* 314 (1986):1226–32.

Devesa, S.S., W.J. Blot, B.J. Stone, B.A. Miller, R.E. Tarone, and J.F. Fraumeni, Jr. Recent cancer trends in the United States. *Journal of the National Cancer Institute* 87, 3 (1995):175–82.

Frey, C.M., M.M. McMillen, C.D. Cowan, J.W. Horm, and L.G. Kessler. Representatives of the surveillance, epidemiology and end results program data: recent trends in cancer mortality rate. *Journal of the National Cancer Institute* (1992):872–77.

McGinnis, J.M. and W.H. Foege. Actual causes of death in the United States. *Journal of the American Medical Association* 270 (1993):2207–12.

Muurinen, J.M. The economics of informal care. Labor market effects in the National Hospice Study. *Medical Care* 24 (1986):1007–17.

Rennie, J., and Rusting. Making headway against cancer. *Scientific American* 275 (1996):28–30.
Walter, S.D., S.E. Birnie, L.D. Marrett, S.M. Taylor, D. Reynolds, J. Davies, J.J. Drake, and M. Hayes. The geographic variation of cancer incidence in Ontario. *American Journal of Public Health* 84, 3 (1994):367–76.

Internet Sources

European Community cancer statistics: http://telescan.nki.nl/iarc.html
SEER cancer statistics: http://www.seer.ims.nci.nih.gov/Publications/ CSR7395/ index.html

Chapter 2

Cancer through the Ages

Our ancestors got cancer. We can see evidence of cancer in prehistoric fossils and in mummies. The earliest medical writings, recorded in the Egyptian Ebers papyrus and the Smith papyrus, contain references to cancer, and they were written about 1600 BC. It is likely that the Smith papyrus is a copy of text written about 2500 BC . The Ebers papyrus, discovered in 1873, was translated successfully in 1937. Its writings do not distinguish between true cancerous tumors and inflammatory swellings. The Smith papyrus is a surgical document, discovered in 1862 and translated in 1922. It describes various surgical conditions, including breast cancer, and it recommends treatments.

Hippocrates (circa 460–370 BC) introduced the term *carcinoma* (in Greek, *karkinoma*, derived from *karkinos*, meaning crab). The claws of the crab symbolized a cancer's tentacles eating into flesh. The crab is still a common symbol for cancer. According to Hippocrates, man contained four basic humors: blood, phlegm, yellow bile, and black bile. When these were mixed in proper proportions we were healthy and when there was an imbalance between them we got disease. This, in reality, was an extension of Aristole's view on nature. Hippocrates postulated that excess black bile caused cancer. He identified two kinds of cancers: (a) malignant ulcers and (b) deep-seated cancers, and described cancer of the skin, cervix, and rectum.

Another Greek, Galen (circa 150 AD), built on Hippocrates's theory that cancer was caused by black bile (*melan cholas*) circulating through the body. This evil substance, he said, was then deposited in various tissues and continued to grow relentlessly. This idea remained, it appears, unchallenged for more than a thousand years. Galen was one of the most influential physicians of all time. Although born in Asia Minor, he spent much of his professional life in Rome. His views controlled medical thinking in the western world for some 1,300 years, until the late Middle Ages. Galen's black bile theory implied that cancer was a systemic disease and should be treated systematically rather than locally. He recommended that diet and purging be added to the treatment. He also distinguished between cancer and nontumorous swellings. During this time both Christianity and Islam frowned on anatomical dissection. The alchemist Paracelsus (1493–1541) put forward another popular theory. He stated that excess mineral salts in the blood, deposited and concentrated at sites of disease, caused cancer.

Andreas Vesalius, professor of anatomy in Padua, wrote the first accurate anatomy text in 1543—*De Humani Corporis Fabrica* (On the Construction of the Human Body). He failed to find a trace of black bile and debunked Galen's theory. He also discovered from his detailed anatomic studies that Galens' published anatomical descriptions were often wrong. He concluded that Galenic human anatomy was not, in fact, based on human dissection, but on dissections of dogs, monkeys, or pigs. The Romans of Galen's time also prohibited dissection of the human body.

In 1628 William Harvey, an English physician who studied anatomy in Padua, discovered how blood circulated through the human body and published *De Motu Cordis* (On the Motion of the Heart). Hildanus (1560–1634), the father of early German surgery, dissected axillary (armpit) lymph nodes for breast cancer. He was the first surgeon to do this operation, which is now standard procedure for many types of breast cancer. As interest in anatomy and dissection grew, the lymph theory took hold. According to it, the cause of cancer was coagulable degenerating lymph, derived from blood, which grew into tumors.

Henry François Le Drun (1685–1770) had remarkable insight into the nature of cancer. He believed that in its early stage cancer was a localized disease and could be cured by early surgery. He believed that breast cancer spread via lymphatics to axillary lymph nodes. Then if a drop of "cancer lymph" passed the lymph nodes it contaminated the entire system.

The black bile, the alchemy, and the lymph theories were remarkably similar and implied that cancer was a systemic disease caused by circulating evil substances deposited at sites of tumor formation. These concepts in some ways reflect our present ideas, as we will see in later chapters. Substitute malignant cells for other traveling evils, and our idea of cancer spread is remarkably similar to those in vogue about 200 AD and throughout the Middle Ages. These theories were all the more remarkable when you consider that the microscope had not yet been invented and all theories were based on naked-eye observations.

In 1761 Giovanni Battista Morgagni published "On the Sites and Causes of Disease," in which he correlated postmortem findings with the clinical records of 700 patients. He described many cancers and clearly separated tumorous neoplasms from other swellings. By then the optical microscope had been invented. Soon its applications contributed to a broadening of knowledge in all the biological fields. For the first time doctors could study cells. Anton van Leeuwenhoek, a Dutch scientist, discovered

red blood cells, bacteria, and protozoa and described the microscopic appearance of muscle. Marcello Malpighi, the most famous microscopist of the seventeenth century, had earlier described the development of chick embryos and was the first to discover capillaries (the tiny blood vessels linking arteries with veins). Leeuwenhoek realized that capillaries completed the circulation of blood theorized by Harvey.

Müller, with the aid of the microscope, established in 1838 that cancers were made of cells and not from coagulated lymph or other fluids. However, he thought that cancer cells arose from "amorphous germinal elements" dispersed between normal tissues. This was the blastema theory of cancer.

Rudolf Virchow (1821–1902), the father of cellular pathology, had studied under Müller and recognized that all normal cells arise from other cells (*omnis cellulae cellula*) and not from amorphous blastema. This cellular theory was soon applied to cancer. He proposed that cancer was caused by chronic irritation in a host with some constitutional or hereditary predisposition. Again, this concept is very close to current teaching. Karl von Rokitansky had earlier proposed the hereditary predisposition theory.

Although he correctly identified the cellular nature of cancer, Virchow thought that bad fluid circulating through the primary tumor caused metastases at distal sites. He failed to appreciate that metastases were caused by circulating tumor cells. Thiersch (1822–1895) recognized that metastases were due to small fragments of tumor breaking off and traveling to distant sites (tumor embolization). We now know that metastases are usually caused by the spread of single cells rather than by hunks of broken-off tumor. Nevertheless, it appears that sometimes tumor cells traveling in small clusters also cause metastases.

Toward the end of the nineteenth century and early in the twentieth century, theories on the causation of cancer included the embryonal theory. The embryonal theory stated that persistent groups of embryonic cells, the remnants of fetal tissue, somehow or other were activated to become malignant as a result of a change in their blood supply. Another popular theory of the time was the mechanical isolation and traumatic origin theory. According to it, multiple small injuries or one major injury could free groups of cells from the restraints of normal surrounding tissue. These free cells then grew uncontrolled to become malignant tumors.

The parasitic theory held that cancer was caused by some infectious agent, and this infectious theory implied that cancer was contagious. This theory was popular in the seventeenth and eighteenth centuries and persisted into the nineteenth and early twentieth centuries. Since most people feared that cancer was contagious, early cancer hospitals functioned somewhat like quarantine units. The first cancer hospital, La Lutte contre le Cancer of Rheims, France, was forced to move out of the city in 1779 because the public was afraid that they might catch cancer from the inmates. Relatives and families, shamed by having cancer in the family, went to great lengths of hide the truth. In many areas of the western world this attitude persisted up to the 1960s. In 1887 Scheurlen isolated a bacillus from breast cancer and claimed to have induced tumors in dogs with this organism. In 1913 Johannes Fibriger claimed that a nematode (a class of worm) caused gastric cancer. Subsequently, he received a Nobel prize in medicine and physiology (1926) for work that has never been verified. During this time period there were many other claims for infectious causes. Rous in 1911 showed that animal sarcomas (cancer of muscle and connective tissue) could be transmitted to other animals by a cell-free filtrate (a virus). Likewise, in 1936 Bittner demonstrated that a filtrable agent (now known to be a retrovirus) could cause breast cancer in mice. As we shall see later, with a few notable exceptions, we still have very little evidence that viruses cause human cancer (unlike many animal cancers).

The optical microscope and later the electron microscope let scientists investigate the structure of cancer in great detail. These instruments also let investigators study the progression from normal cells to abnormal (dysplastic) cells and finally into malignant cells.

Cancer research in the first half of this century focused on its cellular origin. The predominant research tool of the time, the microscope, offered little help in addressing key questions relating to tumor behavior. Since then research has switched to understanding tumor cell behavior. First, there was an emphasis on biochemical techniques. However, for the past twenty-five years our attention has focused on genetic abnormalities within the tumor cell and on how signals from mutant genes direct cell behavior. New sophisticated molecular biological techniques allow us to address questions relating to normal and tumor cell behavior.

Bibliography

Fisher, E.R., and C.M. Hermann. Historic milestones in cancer pathology. *Seminars in Oncology* 6, 4 (1979):428–32.

Hill, G.J., 2d. Historic milestones in cancer surgery. *Seminars in Oncology* 6, 4 (1979): 409–27.

Petrakis, N.L. Historic milestones in cancer epidemiology. *Seminars in Oncology* 6, 4 (1979): 433–44.

Skipper, H.E. Historic milestones in cancer biology: A few that are important in cancer treatment (revised). *Seminars in Oncology* 6, 4 (1979):506–14.

Sournia, J.C. *Histoire de la médecine et des médecins. The illustrated history of medicine.* London: Harold Starke, 1992.

Wold, W.S., and M. Green. Historic milestones in cancer virology. *Seminars in Oncology* 6, 4 (1979):461–78.

CHAPTER 3

Tissue Organization and Differentiation

What is cancer? Before we can begin to answer this question, we need some background information on normal cells and tissues. Brain, heart, lung, skin, and other organs interconnect and communicate with each other through a network of blood vessels, lymphatics, and nerves in a highly sophisticated human machine. We use the term *tissue* in a nonspecific way to describe the arrangement of cells in each organ, e.g., "lung tissue" or "breast tissue." Under the microscope we see that all tissues show certain similarities but also major differences.

A great number of cells reside and grow in harmony in every organ. The cell is the basic building block of every tissue and every organ (figure 3.1). It resembles a room, with its four walls, a ceiling, and a floor; these are the cell membranes. Cells can have different shapes, from cuboidal to spherical and many transitional forms in between. Cells often change their shape. Like a room with doors and windows, cells have openings in their walls that allow movement between neighboring cells. Each cell has a curious machine sitting on its floor—the nucleus. The nucleus contains a rope-like tangle of protein called chromatin. Within this are the chromosomes, and genes are embedded along the chromosomes.

The nucleus acts like a supercomputer. Its purpose is to control the cell's every function. The power of the nucleus resides in one chemical—DNA. This remarkable chemical controls all life on this planet, not just human lives but those of large animals, small animals, insects, and plants. In fact, DNA controls the biological behavior of all living organisms. It is the substance from which genes are made. Each human nucleus contains 100,000 genes; these are not visible with a microscope, not even with an electron microscope. We need new molecular biology tools to see them. (The structure of the gene is discussed in more detail in chapter 8).

A tiny bag of enzyme-enriched fluid, the cytoplasm, surrounds each nucleus. Cytoplasmic organelles (cell components), called ribosomes, and

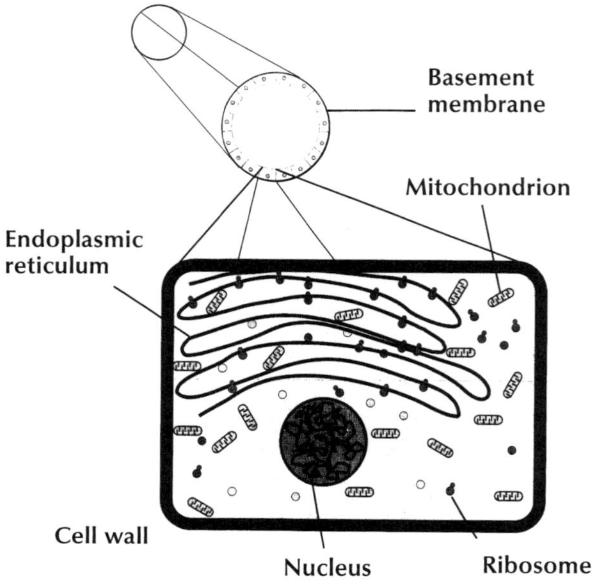

Figure 3.1. *Schematic representation of a normal cell, taken from the lining of any epithelial-lined tissue. (For simplicity, a number of less well known organelles have been omitted.)*

endoplasmic reticulum manufacture proteins, fats, carbohydrates, hormones, and a constellation of chemicals necessary for normal cell function. Genes orchestrate and control the production and movement of these chemicals. Mitochondria provide energy (fuel) for all metabolic and synthetic activity. A semipermeable membrane encloses each nucleus and each of the cytoplasmic organelles. Finally, each cell, with its nucleus and cytoplasm, is surrounded by a cell membrane, like the outer wall of a building.

Despite the striking similarity of all cells to each other, microscopically each tissue is readily recognizable as belonging to a heart, brain, skin, or kidney. Every cell in the body resembles every other cell in that each contains an identical set of genes locked within a nucleus, surrounded by cytoplasm and an outer cell membrane. Cells in each tissue or organ also show subtle differences, reflecting their specialized structure and function. City buildings might be composed of identical bricks. Nevertheless, we identify houses, office blocks and department stores without any difficulty. Their shape, their size, and the way they are put together make them instantly recognizable. So too, microscopic architecture lets us identify each organ. For example, in the skin, cells arrange themselves into distinct layers; squamous (pavementlike) cells in the outer layer (the epidermis) provide protection from the environment, whereas cells in the deeper layers provide nutrition and support for the outer layer. The lining of the mouth and other tissues also contain very similar squamous cells. However, hair follicles and sweat glands are unique to skin, making them readily recognizable and easily distinguished from other squamous-lined tissues.

The process whereby cells develop specialized functions and arrange themselves into specific tissue types is called differentiation. Such differentiation allows brains to think and hearts to pump. The heart pumps five liters of blood around our bodies every minute and its pulsating muscle cells need a lot of energy to do this. Mitochondria, the powerhouses of the cell, are abundant in cells requiring large amounts of energy. As you might expect, other muscles also have abundant mitochondria. In contrast, the skin's main function is to protect the underlying tissues from the hostile environment. Therefore, the outer squamous cells of the skin (keratinocytes) contain an abundance of a tough protective structural protein called keratin and relatively few cytoplasmic mitochondria.

In the differentiating embryo, lymphocytes form garrisons throughout the body; these are the lymph nodes. They function like crack commando outfits, their lymphocytes always at the ready to react immediately to invaders by pouring antibodies and immune-primed lymphocytes into the circulation. Consider what happens when a trivial cut becomes infected. Within the lymphatic and vascular channels, white blood cells guard and protect the tissues they patrol. They rush to any site of infection, exit the bloodstream, and throw a cordon around the invader.

Different white cells have different duties. Neutrophils (polymorphonuclear leukocytes, PMNs) fire a barrage of destructive enzymes at the enemy. At the same time, lymphocytes (our immune cells) secrete deadly chemicals (cytokines) and antibodies. Their comrades, the monocytes or macrophages, are the scavengers. They digest the dead enemy and remove injured tissue. This is what happens in the healthy individual. These cells owe their protective behavior to the process of differentiation. However, sometimes the process does not have such a happy ending. If the invaders, e.g., bacteria, are well protected by their outer coats of biological armor, they may resist and overcome the white cells. This happens with infection by certain virulent organisms. Alternatively, if there are few circulating white cells or if they are damaged by chemotherapy, AIDS (Acquired Immune Deficiency Syndrome), or cancer, they may not put up such a good fight. The result is overwhelming infection and death.

Tissue differentiation begins during the first few hours or days of embryonic life. By the third week of development, cells from three distinct embryonic layers: ectoderm, mesoderm, and endoderm. They divide rapidly and differentiate into the bodys' highly complex and organized tissues.

Ectoderm differentiates into skin, breast, brain, spinal cord, and nerves. The lungs and intestines originate from the endoderm. Muscle, bones, joints, and connective tissue develop from mesoderm. Most organs and tissues have components derived from more than one embryonic layer. Throughout life, tissues remain organized as at birth; for most tissue this differentiation is complete long before birth. In fact, in a normal forty-week pregnancy, organs are well formed and their tissues differentiated after twelve weeks of gestation.

A group of undifferentiated cells, arising from the fertilized egg, form the embryo. As these cells divide and replicate, differentiation genes control the formation of all organs and tissues. Although all cells contain the same genes, different groups are activated or deactivated according to the tissues the cells reside in. For example, in muscle cells the genes responsible for muscle fiber formation are activated or "expressed," while genes responsible for mucus secretion lie dormant and inactive. In the epithelial cells lining the intestine, genes responsible for mucus secretion are active. Those responsible for cleansing the blood and secreting urine lie dormant; these genes are active in kidney cells. However, we still have little under-

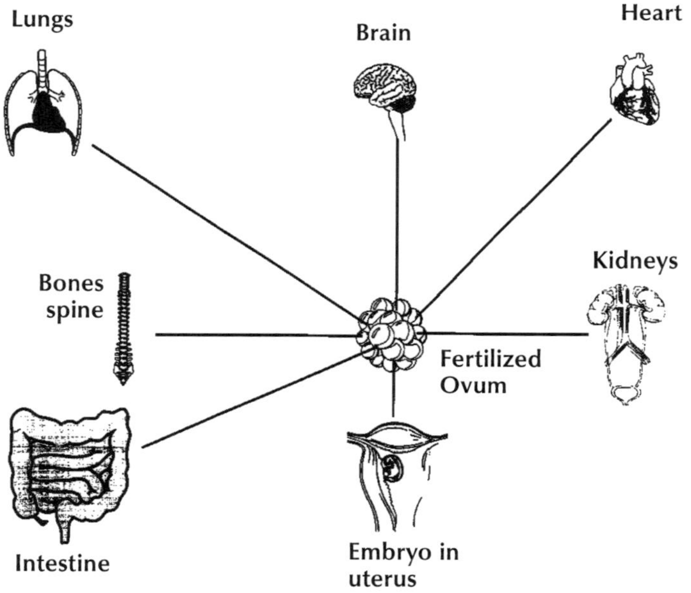

Figure 3.2. Tissue and organ differentiation.

standing of which genes tell which cells they should become colon, kidney, or muscle cells.

During embryonic development, tissues split, fuse, move about, fold, and mold themselves into arms, legs, liver, heart, and other organs. At the same time individual cells differentiate into skin, muscle, brain, and the hundreds of other specialized cells that populate different tissues. In some tissues—for example, bone marrow—a small population of stem cells lie unobtrusively in the background. They retain the ability to proliferate and differentiate if the need ever arises. They generate new marrow in response to cell damage. As we will see in chapter 11, they provide a lifesaving supply of new bone marrow and blood cells for some cancer patients on intensive chemotherapy.

Cancer cells lose the ability to differentiate and function normally. Recent research on early fetal development has also yielded some significant insights into the biology of cancer. Part of the process of fetal sculpting and remodeling is the selective loss of groups of cells by a process called apoptosis. The word is derived from the Greek *apoptos* meaning to drop off; just as dead leaves drop from a tree. Apoptosis is a form of physiologically programmed cell death, popularly known as cell suicide. Apoptotic cells have a distinct and characteristic appearance in the electron microscope. These changes are quite different from those seen in cells killed by poisons or disease. They also show characteristic biochemical changes. Specific suicide genes control apoptosis. Although the process in humans is still not fully understood, one gene known as bcL2 plays a major role. Activation of bcL2 prolongs cell survival and programs cancer cells to live much longer than normal cells, allowing cancer cells to accumulate. This is unlike the situation in most normal tissue, where cells stop growing, die, and are replaced by new cells. Another important gene controlling apoptosis is p53 (discussed in chapter 8). Much of our information on apoptosis has come from studies on the growth and development of a worm called *caenorhabditis elegans.* This creature generates 1090 cells (exactly) and kills 131 cells, to make itself. Fourteen separate genes cooperate to control apoptosis in that worm. In humans, many more genes control apoptosis, and our understanding of apoptosis is still at a rudimentary stage. The relevance of apoptosis to cancer is that some tumors have high apoptotic rates and some have low rates, and some chemotherapeutic drugs exert part of their action by altering apoptosis. Oncologists and patients would welcome any treatment capable of inducing cell suicide in tumors.

While cells grow, divide, die, and are replaced by new cells, the overall organization of each tissue remains the same. The life cycle of individual cells often varies considerably from tissue to tissue. Brain cells (neurons) do not multiply after birth. We lose some neurons as part of the normal aging process. Others are killed off by injury, disease, or alcohol. At the opposite extreme, bone marrow cells and the cells lining our intestines are renewed every few days. Most cells have a life cycle somewhere between these extremes. Many cells can adapt to injury and, if necessary, grow more rapidly to replace dead or damaged cells. The cancer cell has a severely disrupted life cycle.

What controls the miracle of differentiation and tissue organization? We do not yet understand the precise details. However, modern molecular biology provides new clues. Within each nucleus, genes, strung out along our chromosomes, determine our color and gender and how each cell functions. They also determine which cells are destined to become brain cells, which are destined to function as heart cells, and so forth. They control the rate at which each cell divides, grows, and matures. In essence, they control our anatomy, our physiology, and our biochemistry. Some would argue that they also control much of our psychology and behavior. They also initiate and control the progression of cancer. Although embryologists, in the past, studied in great detail the progression of fetal development and differentiation, they did not understand what controlled this magic process. At last they are beginning to identify families of genes responsible for development and differentiation. These are known as homeobox genes (HOX genes). Ed Lewis, from the California Institute of Technology, Pasadena, was awarded the Nobel Prize in 1995 for his work in this area. He used the humble fruit fly to provide many answers about embryonic development. The same genes that control the growth of wings and limbs in the fruit fly control the limbs of mice and men. Mutated HOX genes cause congenital (present at birth) deformities of the hands and skull. Researchers studying the genetic control of differentiation are only at the beginning of their journey. If homeobox genes control normal differentiation, could they also control tumor differentiation? It appears so. We can expect an information explosion in this field of study during the next decade. One of the pathological hallmarks of cancer is abnormal differentiation, and homeobox genes are mutated in many cancers, including cancer of the lung, colon, and kidney. It is easy to speculate that in the future, some form of gene therapy might be successful in restoring a cancer cell's ability to differentiate correctly and change back to a normal cell.

Many of the most exciting recent discoveries have been made by scientists working not directly on cancer but on the basic mechanisms of normal and abnormal cell growth and division. Since cancer occurs in our biological cousins 50 and even 500 million years distant on the evolutionary timeline, we should not be surprised that yeasts, fruit flies, worms, mice, and rats all contribute to a new understanding of cancer.

Our environment, what we breathe, and what we eat also play a major role in how we function. However, even environmental changes are monitored and modulated by our genes. We are the product of our genes and their interaction with the environment. Except for our red blood cells (which carry oxygen to all our tissues) and platelets (which prevent us from bleeding to death by forming blood clots at sites of minor injury), all cells contain at least one nucleus. Remarkably, every nucleus contains the same genes. Even more remarkably, different sets of genes are switched on or off in genes of the liver, heart, or some other organ. Genes in the heart instruct myocytes (muscle cells) to produce contractile filaments, called actin and myosin. These act in harmony, contracting and relaxing with each heartbeat. In the kidney, a different set of genes instruct cells to produce the complex biochemical machinery required to purify the bloodstream and remove waste products. Although kidney cells have the same complement of muscle-producing genes as myocytes, these genes lie dormant and inactive. The detailed mechanisms controlling switching on (promoters) and switching off (inhibitors) of different sets of genes are still a mystery; however, we know that these switches are also genes.

This brief description of cell structure, differentiation, and their genetic control (discussed in more detail in chapter 8) provides some background for our understanding of the cellular abnormalities in cancer.

In essence, cancer results from the continued proliferation and accumulation of abnormal cells, due to loss of normal cell growth regulation. In view of the essential role that genes play in regulating normal growth and differentiation, we should not be surprised then to find that genes play a critical role in the development of cancer. Cancer is a genetic disease; it is caused by damaged, malfunctioning genes. Sometimes the damage is inherited. More often it is acquired, the result of some environmental carcinogen acting on susceptible genes. For many cancers this susceptibility may be inherited.

Bibliography

Cory, S. Fascinating death factor. *Science* 367: 317–18.

Cotran, R.S., V. Kumar, and S.L. Robbins. *Robbins pathologic basis of disease.* Philadelphia: Saunders, 1994.

Kerr, J.F.R., C.M. Winterford, and B.V. Harmon. Apoptosis: Its significance in cancer and cancer therapy. *Cancer* 73 (1994):2013–26.

Kerr, J.F.R., A.H. Wyllie, and A.R. Currie. Apoptosis: A basic biological phenomenon with wide-ranging implications in tissue kinetics. *British Journal of Cancer* 26 (1972):239–57.

Majno, G., and I. Joris. *Cells: tissues, and disease: principles of general pathology.* Cambridge, Mass.: Blackwell Science, 1996.

Rubin, E., and J.L. Farber. *Pathology.* Philadelphia: J.B. Lippincott, 1994.

Salomon, R.N., and S. Diaz-Caño. Introduction to apoptosis. *Diagnostic Molecular Pathology* 4 (1995):235–38.
Schumtz, S.M., and M.R. Bennett. Death by any other name. *American Journal of Pathology* 147 (1995):229–43.
Sharpe, P. HOX gene mutations—The wait is over. *Nature Medicine* 2, 7 (1996): 748–49.
Steller, H. Mechanisms and genes of cellular suicide. *Science* 267, 5203 (1995): 1445–49.
Wyllie, A.H. Apoptosis. Death gets a brake. *Nature* 369, 6478 (1994):272–73.
Young, S. Life and death in the condemned cell. *New Scientist* 25 (1992):34–37.

Chapter 4

The Cell's Response to Stress

Imagine a weed growing in a perfectly manicured lawn, in a neighborhood of perfect lawns. This lawn has been neglected for four weeks. Shortly after the owner goes away on a long summer vacation, a few weeds appear. At first, they put down roots and grow slowly in one particular part of the lawn that has little sunlight and poor drainage. If not eradicated quickly, scruffy weeds spread rapidly out of control and strangle the luscious green grass. Before the lawn is destroyed, it is likely that some seeds will blow into nearby and distant gardens. Some of the neighbors' lawns will resist such invaders. Others will succumb to varying degrees.

To prevent such a horticultural catastrophe, a knowledgeable gardener will destroy the first weeds by "surgically" removing them along with their deep roots or by poisoning them with weed killer. A variety of maneuvers—such as weeding, using appropriate weed killer, and reseeding or transplanting grass from a nearby normal area—may revive the lawn. However, imagine a scenario where the remnants of incompletely removed weeds become resistant to all chemicals and continue to proliferate, spread, and destroy the neighbors' lawns.

This scenario is somewhat analogous to cancer. Remove cancer early and everything will be fine. After cancer has spread, eradication is more difficult and the cancer may become resistant to chemotherapy. However, the analogy is imperfect. Unlike the lawn, which needs continuous cutting and maintenance, the body and its tissues are self-regulating, provided that they get a continuous supply of normal nutrients. It might be that soon genetically manipulated lawn grass may seldom need cutting. Already we have the genetically engineered tomato. Apart from hair and nails, human tissues do not need regular trimming. However, let's stay with the weed analogy for a while and use it to explain one particular cancer, malignant melanoma.

Melanocytes are normal melanin-producing skin cells; melanin is what

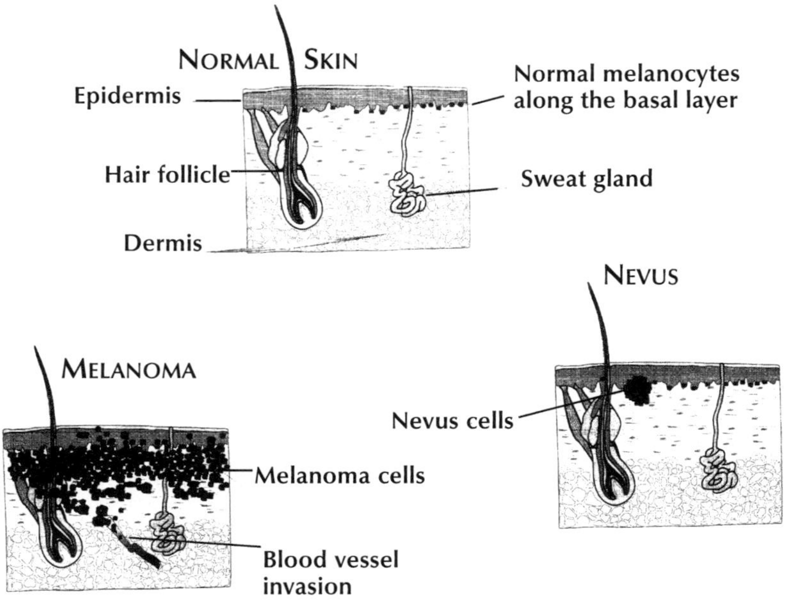

Figure 4.1. Benign nevus and malignant melanoma.

makes dark skin dark. They sit along the lower layer of the skin layer, called the epidermis (figure 4.1). When they collect into groups, they produce an innocent pigmented mole, a benign tumor. This is a nevus. Most of us have one or more benign nevi scattered over our bodies. They usually remain harmless and unnoticed throughout our lives. The cancerous counterpart of the nevus is the malignant melanoma, a potentially lethal form of cancer. It too begins unnoticed, as a small dark patch or bump on the skin that is composed of melanocytes. Unlike the harmless mole, it grows relentlessly, often slowly, but sometimes quickly, changing its color insidiously to various shades of brown-black. The growing melanoma's edge becomes irregular and no longer has the sharp, even border characteristic of a nevus. Beneath the visible surface, its tentacle-like roots, composed of malignant tumor cells, penetrate the deep layer of the skin (the dermis). At some stage, as it burrows downward, tumor cells crawl into small lymphatic channels and blood vessels. These channels are conduits to distal organs. Just as the weeds scatter and take hold in the neighbors' lawns and gardens, so too, melanoma cells spread to local and distant organs—lymph nodes (lymph glands), lungs, brain, and liver. Here they continue to grow at an ever-increasing rate. They eventually destroy these tissues and kill the patient.

Despite its lethal potential, melanoma is curable. Early diagnosis and surgery is curative in most patients, provided that surgery removes the cancer before its roots penetrate the lymphatics and blood vessels. Removing the tumor after it has metastasized to distant sites is like closing the door after the horse has bolted. Melanoma, for example, is a type of cancer that usually resists all forms of chemotherapy and radiotherapy; and immunotherapy is rarely helpful. Could it be that we can also cure other lethal cancers by early diagnosis and treatment? Unequivocally, the answer is yes.

The key abnormality in cancer is uncontrolled cell growth. Normal cells grow in a highly organized, programmed fashion. As tissues grow, differentiate, and maintain their normal structure, cells talk to their neighbors. Each cell knows how often it has to divide. It knows that when it touches a nearby cell it must halt. It must stay in its own preordained position; it must not encroach on its neighbor's space. This property by which cells stop dividing and proliferating when they touch adjacent cells is called *contact inhibition*. Dozens of chemical signals trigger cell growth and harmonize cell-to-cell interactions. Such signals come from growth or suppressor factors, and messages coming from our genes control these chemicals.

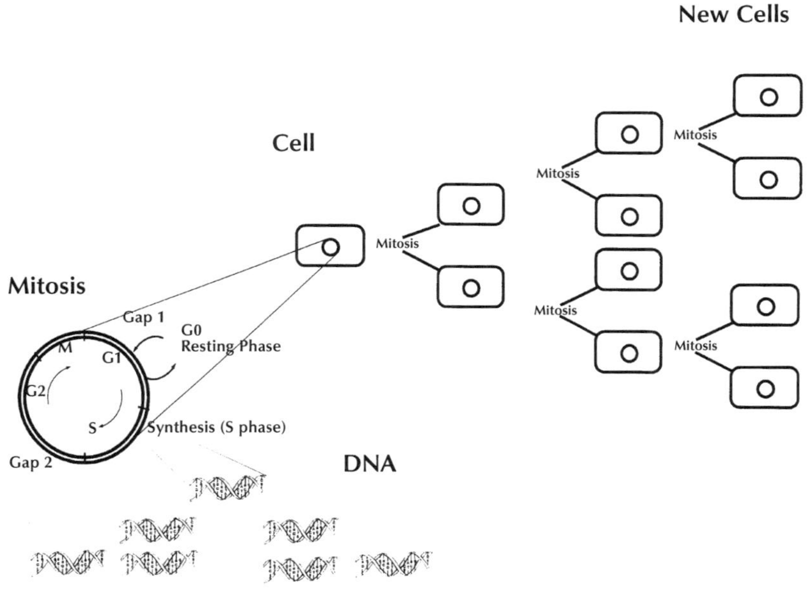

Figure 4.2. *Cell cycle and mitosis.*

Dividing cells pass through a cell cycle. The various phases of the cycle have specific names (figure 4.2.). At any one time most cells are not actively dividing; they are in a resting phase called G0 (G zero). Some cells spend their entire lives locked in G0. The large, specialized, thinking neurons in our brains let us sense our environment and control muscle movement; they work at a tremendous rate. However, they do not divide or multiply. The opposite side of the coin to G0 is the mitotic phase, or the M phase. Each cell, during mitosis, divides and produces two identical daughter cells. Between these phases there are two gap phases, G1 and G2, and a very important S phase. During the synthesis (S) phase, nuclear DNA replicates and migrates to opposite poles of the cell in readiness for the mitotic division. During the G1 and G2 phases, cellular enzymes, proteins, and regulators necessary for cell division accumulate in preparation for the cell division.

The cell cycle can be summarized in shorthand as passing through the G0, G1, S, G2, and M phases and then returning to G0. We can categorize tissues according to their rate of cell proliferation. For convenience sake, we use three categories, labile, stable, and permanent. Labile cells are constantly dividing and renewing themselves, sometimes as quickly as every twenty-four hours, or even quicker. Good examples are bone-marrow cells, immune cells (lymphocytes), and cells lining the intestinal tract and the outer surface of the skin. The stable cells sit happily and carry out their work at a calm and constant pace unless something irritates, stimulates, or injures them. Liver cells are an example of stable cells, and they carry an enormous workload. We carry 1.5 kg of liver cells (hepatocytes) in our upper abdomen. They make protein, synthesize coagulation factors to stop us from hemorrhaging, excrete breakdown products from the metabolism of bile, and protect us by detoxifying drugs or toxins we might ingest. Under normal physiological conditions, liver cells do not divide very frequently; some investigators estimate they divide about once a year. However, if you remove a piece of liver, or poison some liver cells, the liver immediately switches programs and goes into a construction mode. Remarkably, the excised portion of liver will quickly replenish itself with new liver cells. Liver cells, although normally stable and nondividing, can proliferate when required to do so. Just as remarkable as the production of new liver tissue is the way it molds itself to produce an identical replica of the removed tissue. (We will return to discuss permanent cells later.)

The cell cycle holds many of cancer's secrets, and gradually biologists are identifying them. If we knew exactly what controls led each phase of the cycle, perhaps we could modify the cycle to inhibit or stop cell growth. In fact, despite huge gaps in our knowledge, we already know much about this remarkable cycle. Pharmacologists design drugs to deactivate various enzymes controlling the cycle. By combining drugs active at different phases of the cycle, oncologists can successfully eradicate many forms of cancer cells. The biggest problem with such drug combinations is that they also kill rapidly dividing normal cells. What the pharmacologists, oncologists, and patients want is a panel of drugs that will selectively destroy tumor cells and leave normal cells unharmed. No such drugs exist.

Labile and stable cells adapt to injury or to excess biochemical, physiological, or physical stress in different ways. Some stimuli produce benign tissue enlargement. (See figure 4.3). On the left, a hypothetical "unit" of tissue contains nine cells. In response to physical or chemical stress, this unit more than doubles its size by hyperplasia, hypertrophy, or metaplasia. In hyperplasia, the individual cells remain the same size but the total number of cells increases. In hypertrophy, the same degree of unit enlargement occurs, but this time the enlargement is due to increased cell size. In metaplasia, the cells change from one type of cell to another, illustrated here by a change from rectangular (columnar) to spindle-shaped. Metaplastic changes can occur without any tissue enlargement. These three types of change are reversible if the stimulus that causes the change is removed. Growth continues for a limited time or until the tissue reaches a certain size, and then it stops. For example as men grow older their prostate glands enlarge due to an imbalance of hormones, in particular, testosterone. This causes benign prostatic hyperplasia. If the enlargement is considerable it causes urinary obstruction, necessitating surgery.

If you exercise regularly, you get fitter and your muscles get stronger and bigger. Because muscle cells have a poor capacity to divide and proliferate, they respond to increased work by getting larger. Each muscle cell within the biceps or quadriceps—or whatever muscle you exercise—gets bigger or hypertrophied. The sum of the hypertrophied individual muscle fibers adds up to a large muscle mass. The opposite happens if you sit around and do not use your muscles. They waste away; they atrophy. Muscle wasting becomes severe in patients immobilized after traffic accidents. Damage to nerves supplying a muscle also causes muscle atrophy, as is seen in poliomyelitis victims. Muscle responds to physical work by increasing cell size. Other tissues, for example, the thyroid gland, may also respond to stimuli by becoming atrophied or hypertrophied. The stimulus may be a hormone or vitamin or some other chemical.

Another adaptive response is metaplasia. Some cells are better equipped than others to resist a hostile environment. Skin has an outer layer of tough, resistant squamous cells. If the delicate cells lining the lungs are constantly bombarded by noxious cigarette smoke, they respond by altering their structure and they become squamous cells. Squamous cells give better protection against the smoke. However, they lose many of the functions for which

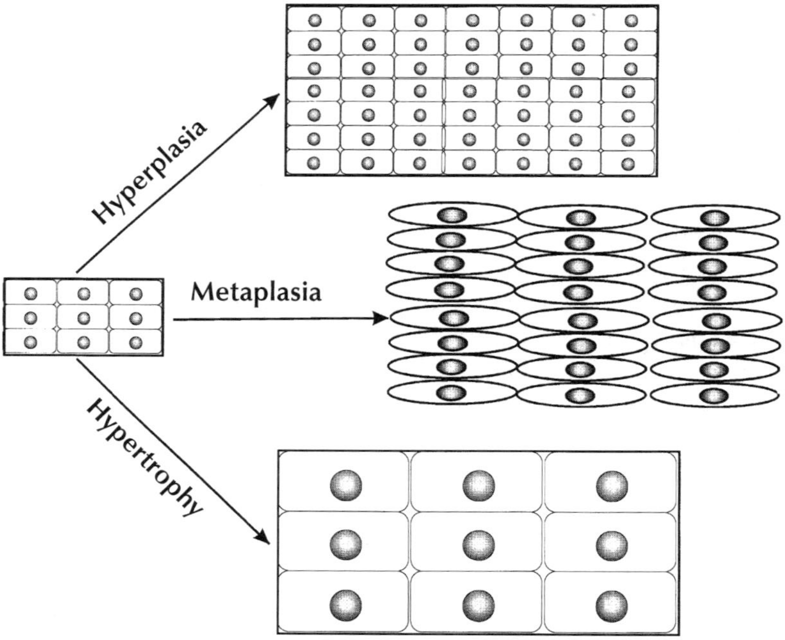

Figure 4.3. Cell response to stress.

lung cells are designed. This process by which one cell type changes to another is called metaplasia. After the injurious stimulus is removed (the patient stops smoking), the cells return to normal.

The third category of cells, permanent cells, have no capacity to regenerate. When they are destroyed, they are replaced by some other form of tissue, usually scar tissue. This happens, for example, after a heart attack. When a blood clot cuts off the coronary blood flow, a segment of heart, deprived of its oxygen supply, dies. The dead tissue is heart muscle. Over a period of six weeks, the dead tissue is removed and replaced by scar tissue. If the scar is small, the patient may live for many years with little or no debility. However, even after twenty or thirty years that scar will continue to occupy part of the heart. Most common cancers arise from labile or stable cells and only rarely from permanent cells.

Hyperplasia, hypertrophy, atrophy, and metaplasia are cellular adaptive mechanisms that are reversible. When the stimulus is changed or removed, altered cells can revert to normal. Malignant cells lose this capacity and they continue to grow and divide, even after the initiating stimulus (such as smoking) is removed. Each cancer cell loses some or many of its normal self-regulating mechanisms. Furthermore, it acquires new powers not available to the normal mature cell. It self-replicates inappropriately, and usually too often. This is due to an inappropriate abundance of growth factors or to a heightened sensitivity to their action. As they lose their self-regulating mechanisms, millions of tumor cells gradually accumulate at one site. In normal tissues, there is a balance between cell gain and cell loss. As tumor cells persist and grow insidiously (remarkably for up to ten years or longer), they eventually form a colony of cells, a bump, visible to the naked eye.

Most cancers begin as a single tumor which, over time, spreads to other tissues. These metastases grow as multiple, coalescing destructive tumors. There is one notable exception—leukemia. While leukemia also begins as a single cell gone wrong, it does not grow as a solid tumor. Leukemia originates in the bone marrow and is a cancer of the white blood cells. These cells fight infection and control our normal immune protective mechanisms. Leukemia cells remain in a fluid form, circulating continuously as single cells in the bloodstream. Eventually they settle, like other cancer cells, in multiple organs, and like other cancer cells they proliferate and grow out of control. Like any other cancer, if it is not treated successfully, leukemia kills.

Bibliography

Albelda, S.M. Role of integrins and other cell adhesion molecules in tumor progression and metastasis. *Laboratory Investigation* 68, 1 (1993):4–17.

Bishop, J.M., and R.A. Weinberg. *Scientific American Molecular Oncology*. New York: Scientific American Medicine, 1996.

Majno, G., and I. Joris. *Cells, tissues, and disease: Principles of general pathology*. Cambridge, Mass.: Blackwell Science, 1996.

Pietenpol, J.A., and B. Vogelstein. Tumor suppressor genes. No room at the p53 inn. *Nature* 365, 6441 (1993):17–18.

Rubin, E., and J. L. Farber. *Pathology*. Philadelphia: J.B. Lippincott, 1994.

Ruoslahti, E. How cancer spreads. *Scientific American* 275 (1996):42–47.

Steller, H. Mechanisms and genes of cellular suicide. *Science* 267, 5203 (1995): 1445–49.

Weinberg, R.A. The cell cycle clock and cancer. *Scientific American* 275 (1996): 36–37.

_____. How cancer arises. *Scientific American* 275 (1996):62–70.

CHAPTER 5

Precancer, Invasion, and Metastases

Many, if not all, cancers evolve over a period of years through a phase called precancer. We use various terms to describe the changes that take place during this interval. *Dysplasia* is the commonest term, and there are varying degrees of dysplasia. Dysplastic cells have abnormal, large, irregular nuclei, a reflection of their abnormal DNA content. An alternative term for *dysplasia* is *nuclear atypia*. The earliest abnormality preceding the growth of all cancers if some form of DNA genetic damage. A hereditary gene mutation can cause this damage. More commonly something in the environment, for example, a chemical or a virus, is the culprit. A tiny amount of DNA damage produces no significant microscopic abnormality in the appearance of the cell. When this cell divides, it passes on the DNA defect to its daughter cells, and these in turn to their daughter cells. This family of altered cells, all with the same DNA abnormality, is called a clone.

In the first cartoon in figure 5.1, one cell changes and becomes dysplastic. This dysplastic cell divides and proliferates, and its offspring are all dysplastic. In time, additional cell abnormalities accumulate and one of the dysplastic cells becomes malignant. As this cell grows and divides it gives rise to a colony of carcinoma cells. Because these are confined above the basement membrane, this is carcinoma in situ. Eventually, the carcinoma cells acquire new properties that allow them to destroy the basement membrane and invade the underlying tissue. One such cell is illustrated at the bottom of the carcinoma in situ. The term *monoclonal* means that all these carcinoma cells originate from one original dysplastic cell. Almost all cancers are monoclonal, whereas most benign tumors and tumorlike growths are polyclonal (originating from many different cells).

Damaged DNA is unstable and prone to cumulative abnormalities during the process of cell division and replication. Gradually, accumulating DNA damage alters the appearance of the nucleus so that it can be recognized microscopically as dysplastic. Usually, this phase takes many years.

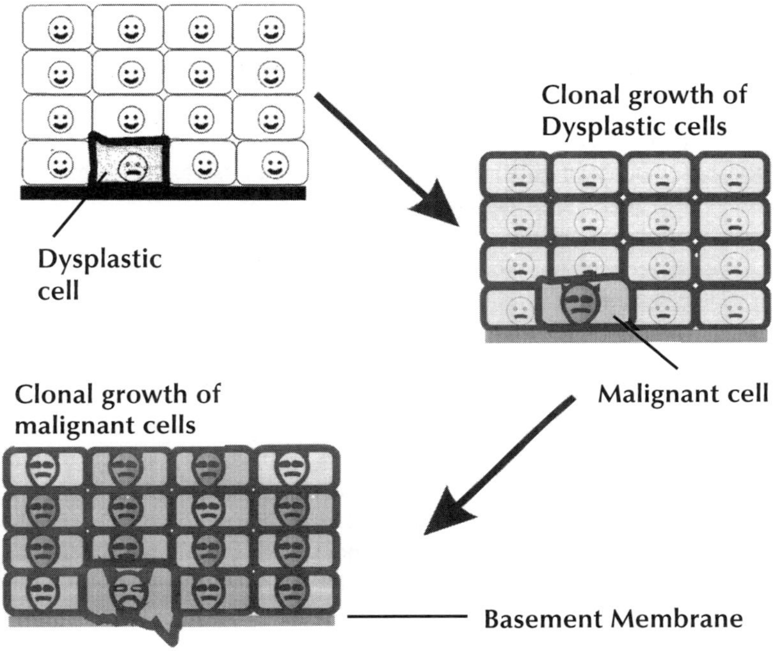

Figure 5.1. Clonal growth of carcinoma in situ (with early invasive change).

Pathologists classify increasing degrees of dysplasia as mild, moderate, and severe, according to how abnormal the cells look under the microscope. The more severe the dysplasia, the closer it is to cancer. Eventually, severe dysplasia evolves into early preinvasive cancer; this is carcinoma in situ. It is possible, and likely, that many cases of mild dysplasia never progress to cancer, but, as it were, self-heal. The clinical importance of dysplasia and carcinoma in situ is that they are totally curable. An intact basement membrane acts as a barrier to cancer cells, and they cannot metastasize until they have broken through this barrier. Once a tumor penetrates the basement membrane it is no longer carcinoma in situ; it is now invasive carcinoma (figure 5.2). Normal cells, on the left, gradually change to dysplastic cells. These are slightly larger and irregular. In particular, nuclei show abnormal contours. The size and nuclear irregularities grow progressively worse as cells become malignant and invade through the basement membrane. In carcinoma in situ, the malignant cells are confined above the basement membrane and cannot metastasize. However, once they have become invasive through the basement membrane they can then penetrate lymphatics and blood vessels and metastasize to distant organs. Carcinoma in situ and its precursors give us a wonderful opportunity to prevent death from cancer. Remove the precursor and you stop the development and progression of the malignancy. This fact provides the rationale for cancer-screening programs.

Normal epithelial cells hold hands and bind tightly to each other and to the basement membrane, using velcrolike hooks called desmosomes. Desmosomes are large enough to see with the aid of an electron microscope. Invisible even to the electron microscope are the thousands of specialized adhesion molecules that are embedded in the outer cell membrane. Adhesion molecules cover the cell surface like a layer of sticky sugar and lightly glue cells to their neighbors. (See figure 5.3). As cells change from normal to dysplastic cells, and then to carcinoma in situ, to invasive carcinoma, and finally to metastases, they accumulate DNA damage and genetic mistakes. Some mistakes affect genes' coding for desmosomes and cell adhesion molecules. As a result, these sticky bits are not produced at all, or if they are, they are made incorrectly. As a result, cells become unstable and fall off the basement membrane from the outer surface of the tumor. Because they are no longer bound tightly to each other, doctors can easily obtain a sample of cells to examine under the microscope by gently scraping or rubbing the tissue surface. This is how they obtain cells for the PAP smear test, which is the cornerstone of cervical cancer screening.

In each tissue, normal cells behave as a community. Signals pass from cell to cell, and, as information is shared, cells know what their neighbors

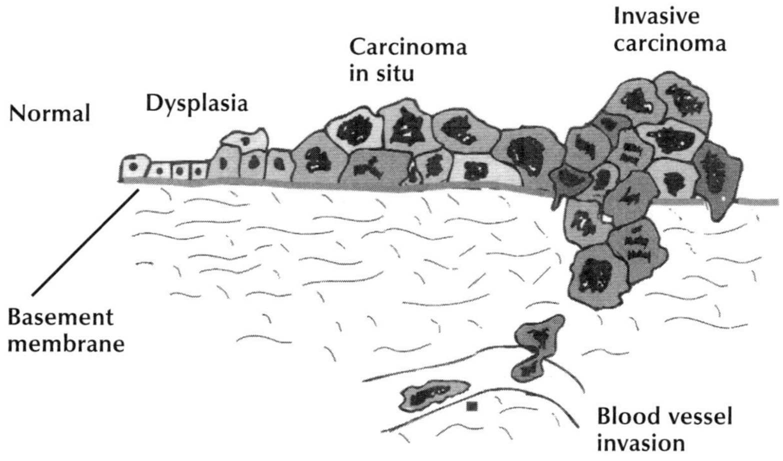

Figure 5.2. Progression of malignant changes.

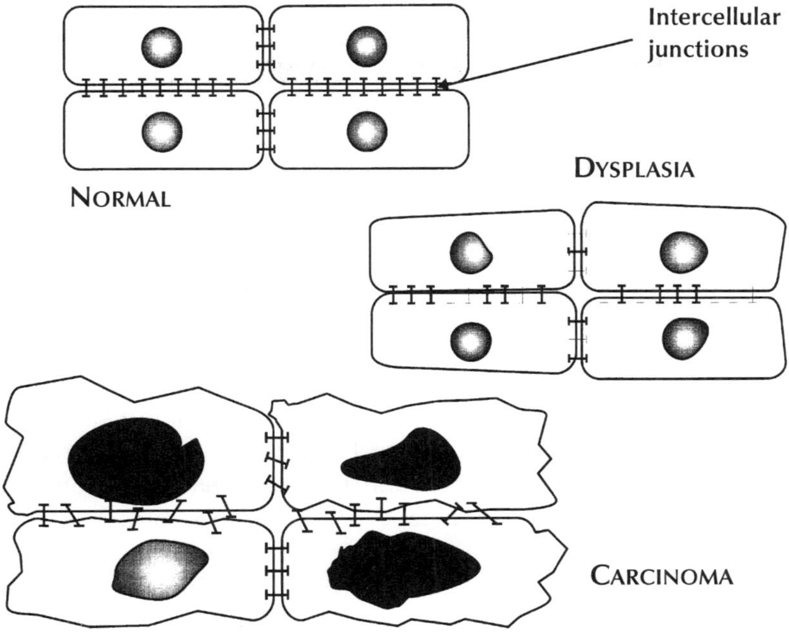

Figure 5.3. Loss of cell adhesion.

are doing. With loss of adhesion comes some loss of cell signaling. Gradually, they become more independent and unruly. Although they lose some normal growth properties, they gain new advantageous properties that allow them to live more independently in their own microcosm. In some ways, the process is analogous to accelerated evolution. Selfish genes provide their malignant cells with the structure and biochemical properties necessary to evolve independently and to grow and spread and eventually take over the entire body. Some patients visualize cancer cells as science-fiction-like aliens taking over and conquering their bodies. Ultimately, however, the process is self-defeating and worse than a Pyrrhic victory. When the tumor has finally won its battle and killed its host, it too must die. Others see cancer as parasites moving about their bodies, ingesting their food and vitamins and leaving them malnourished and wasted.

Most primary tumors do not kill patients, since they can be removed successfully by surgery or radiotherapy. Metastases kill. Many researchers focus on the events contributing to metastases. In order to metastasize, tumors must penetrate basement membranes and invade blood or lymphatic vessels. After metastasizing they must survive and grow like their primary progenitors. What molecular events confer on the cancer cells the power to metastasize? The more we delve into the mechanics of the cell cycle, cell proliferation, apoptosis, differentiation, and angiogenesis (blood vessel information) the more we realize that most of these processes are intimately linked by a web of chemical signals continuously sampling and responding to changes elsewhere on the vascular network.

How do tumors metastasize? An envelope called a basement membrane surrounds normal epithelial cells, such as those of the skin or those lining internal organs. During the early stages of tumor growth the basement membrane acts as a growth barrier, protecting surrounding connective tissue, lymphatics, and blood vessels. Among a cancer cell's newly acquired properties is its ability to become motile. Somewhat like the unicellular amoebae it changes shape and moves through cracks and crevices in the basement membrane. It can also secrete destructive enzymes that knock holes in the membrane. Holes in the basement membrane allow malignant cells to squeeze through the barrier. Once they have escaped into the connective tissue, they seek and destroy other basement membranes surrounding and protecting capillaries and tiny veins. They now enter the circulation and travel to draining lymph nodes and distant organs.

Researchers in laboratories worldwide are investigating which genes control these mechanisms. They are trying to find out what switches on and off the controlling genes. They believe that a comprehensive understanding of the processes may open avenues for some new forms of therapy.

After malignant cells have breached the basement membrane, they must make their way through the surrounding connective tissue matrix. Like almost every other step in cancer initiation and progression, the mechanisms controlling this step are not fully understood. It is likely that some of the mechanisms involved are common to all cancers and some are unique to individual tumors or groups of tumors. The traditional view is that cancer cells dissolve the surrounding matrix, and that surface receptors allow the tumor cells to bind to scaffoldlike proteins as they crawl to the nearest lymphatic or blood vessel.

Besides destroying the host matrix, many tumors make their own stroma, or connective tissues. If you examine a breast carcinoma under the microscope, you will see that often 50 percent or more of the tumor consists of a fibrous stroma. This stromal reaction is common to many cancers. In the past, we assumed that the host tissue made this fibrous component in an attempt to control the spread of tumor cells. We now know that some or much of the tumor stroma is produced by the tumor cells and not by the host. Tumor cells, as well as destroying the host matrix, make their own scaffolding. By producing new stroma, tumor cells favorably condition their own microenvironment with a plethora of chemical signaling agents, nutrients, and growth factors. In this milieu, they thrive and proliferate.

Cancer cells also trick the host tissue into thinking that they are lymphocytes and this metamorphosis allows the malignant cells to metastasize to lymph nodes. How do they do this? Lymphocytes have a receptor called CD44 on their surface. This protein has a complementary receptor in lymph nodes, which sticks to the CD44 and allows normal activated lymphocytes to bind to lymph nodes. Metastatic tumor cells produce a specific type of CD44 to mimic lymphocyte behavior. As they flow in lymphatic fluid, through a lymph node, they stick to the lymph node receptors. Here they stay and grow.

Tumor cells have another useful weapon. They secrete a vascular growth factor, known as tumor angiogenesis factor (TAF). As some cancer clones enlarge, they outgrow their normal blood supply. The center of many rapidly growing tumors dies from oxygen deprivation and lack of nutrition. To overcome this, tumors produce their own blood supply. By secreting TAF and a variety of other chemicals and growth factors, cancer cells stimulate the nearby blood vessels to sprout tiny capillaries, like thousands of tiny branches from the limb of a tree. This process is referred to as tumor neoangiogenesis (new blood vessel formation). Tumor angiogenesis ensures that tumor cells have their own blood supply with oxygen and its life-supporting nutrients.

The process resembles, to some extent, what happens at the site of a cut or wound. Tiny capillaries grow in from the surrounding normal tissue and they carry whatever ingredients are necessary to repair the damaged tissue. If you look closely at a skin wound, you will notice that the surrounding skin is swollen and red and feels hot. It may also throb painfully. This change in the adjacent skin is due to increased blood flow and an increased number of blood vessels at the site of injury. After the injury, a process of healing takes place, capillaries regress, and gradually the appearance returns to normal.

Cancers, however, in their relentless march, continue to produce new blood vessels. Like the accelerators and brakes controlling cell proliferation there is also a constant battle to produce and to inhibit new vessels. Chemical mediators control the flow and ebb of neoangiogenesis. Some of these mediators also cause the capillaries to become leaky, allowing nutrients to seep from the vessels and surround tumor cells. Many biotechnology and pharmaceutical companies see angiogenesis as an opportunity to become rich. By identifying the chemicals responsible for tumor angiogenesis they hope to abolish the actions of these chemicals. A trillion epithelial cells line the blood vessels in a 70kg adult. These stretch over an area of 1,000 square meters, the estimated surface area of the vascular system. Normally these are slow-growing stable cells. When stimulated they proliferate rapidly—as rapidly as bone marrow cells, if necessary—and produce new vessels.

Early, small tumors can grow to approximately 2–3mm^3 (the size of a pinhead) without new blood vessels. Tumors of this size contain about 1 million cells. Tumors larger than this need their own blood supply.

A major medical puzzle is why metastases sometimes lie dormant for years and then become reactivated. Angiogenesis may provide the answer. A recent hypothesis suggests that tiny metastases are in a state of growth equilibrium; the rate of cell growth equals the rate of cell loss by apoptosis. At some stage this equilibrium is upset by the onset of angiogenesis. Once neovascularization is established, the phase of latency is finished and metastases grow and become clinically significant.

Our new knowledge on angiogenesis has diagnostic, prognostic, and therapeutic implications. Using magnetic resonance imaging (MRI), radiologists recognize diagnostic vascular patterns in the brain characteristic of cancer. They are developing similar techniques to diagnose breast cancer and other cancers. Pathologists have found that patient survival is often related to the number of vessels within the tumor. This information may be helpful in identifying patients with a good or bad prognosis. It may also identify those patients more likely to respond to new antiangiogenesis therapy.

Along with the exciting news about tumor angiogenesis came additional information about the cells lining the new vessels. These endothelial cells have distinctive molecules on their surface, molecules that appear to be present in tumor vessels but not in normal vessels. Endoglin and endosialin are two such proteins. Already, the pharmacologists are thinking up methods for targeting these endothelial cells with cytotoxic drugs, antibodies, isotopes, or toxins. The idea is to damage the tumor vessels and starve the tumor of oxygen and nutrients but leave normal blood vessels intact. This field of research has already progressed to early clinical trial phases.

In addition to helping us understand the mechanisms of metastases, the gene scientists have also identified a number of new genes that appear to correlate with the propensity to metastasize. Some of these, such as p53, are involved with cell cycle control. Others may influence different stages of invasion.

Many cancers have defects in the structure of a newly discovered gene, called MTS1 (M stands for multiple). This gene plays a major role in controlling the cell cycle. It monitors and responds to signals arriving in the nucleus from the surrounding cell membrane and cytoplasm. The gene NM23 (NM stands for nonmetastatic), identified in 1988, helps normal cells to differentiate and mature. Loss or malfunction of this gene somehow confers metastatic powers on tumor cells. Experiments on animals show that when NM23 is inserted into tumor cells by genetic manipulation, it blocks the cancer cells from metastasizing. It is likely that many other unidentified genes contribute to metastases. KAI1 is a recently recognized gene on chromosome 11. Like NM23, this gene appears to suppress the metastatic potential of prostate cancer. Loss or damage to KAI1 allows prostate cancer, in animals, to metastasize. Insertion of the normal gene into the experimental tumor cells prevents them from metastasizing. KAI1 is active in some normal human tissues, such as the prostate, lung, liver, and kidney. This suggests that KAI1 may be important in suppressing metastases in many tumor types.

Bibliography

Asa, T., A.O. Borresen, S. Geisler, B. Smith Sorensen, H. Johnsen, J.E. Varhaug, L.A. Akslen, and P.E. Lonning. Specific P53 mutations are associated with de novo resistance to doxorubicin in breast cancer patients. *Nature Medicine* 2, 7 (1996): 811–14.

Akiyama, S.K., K. Olden and K.M. Yamada. Fibronectin and integrins in invasion and metastasis. *Cancer Metastasis Review* 14, 3 (1995):173–89.

Albelda, S.M. Role of integrins and other cell adhesion molecules in tumor progression and metastasis. *Laboratory Investigation* 68, 1 (1993):4–17.

Axelrod, N. Of telomeres and tumors. *Nature Medicine* 2, 2 (1996):158–59.

Bishop, J.M., and R.A. Weinberg. *Scientific American Molecular Oncology*. New York: Scientific American Medicine, 1996.

Cooper, D.L., and G.J. Dougherty. To metastasize or not? Selection of CD44 splice sites. *Nature Medicine* 1 (1995):635–37.

Cotran, R.S., V. Kumar, and S.L. Robbins. *Robbins pathologic basis of disease*. Philadelphia: Saunders, 1994.

Folkman, J. Fighting cancer by attacking its blood supply. *Scientific American* 275 (1996):116–19.

_____. Clinical applications of research on angiogenesis. *New England Journal of Medicine* 333, 26 (1995):1757–63.

Greider, C.W., and E.H. Blackburn. Telomeres, telomerase and cancer. *Scientific American* 274, 2 (1996):92–97.

Harris, C.C., and M. Hollstein. Clinical implications of the p53 tumor-suppressor gene. *New England Journal of Medicine* 329, 18 (1993):1318–27.

Hart, I.R., and A. Saini. Biology of tumour metastasis. *Lancet* 339, 8807 (1992): 1453–57.

Iozzo, R.V. Tumor stroma as a regulator of neoplastic behavior. *Laboratory Investigation* 73 (1995):157–60.

Kamb, A. Cancer. Sun protection factor p53. *Nature* 372, 6508 (1994): 730–31.

Kinzler, K.W., and B. Vogelstein. Cancer therapy meets p53. *New England Journal of Medicine* 331, 1 (1994):49–50.

Lindahl, T. DNA repair. DNA surveillance defect in cancer cells. *Current Biology* 4, 3 (1994):249–51.

Majno, G., and I. Joris. *Cells, tissues, and disease: Principles of general pathology*, Cambridge, Mass.: Blackwell Science, 1996.

Marx, J. DNA repair comes into its own. *Science* 266, 5186 (1994):728–30.

_____. New link found between p53 and DNA repair. *Science* 266, 5189 (1994): 1321–22.

Murray, C. tumor dormancy: not so sleepy after all. *Nature Medicine* 1, 2 (1995): 117–18.

Nabel, G.J., and C. Grunfeld. Calories lost—Another mediator of cancer cachexia? *Nature Medicine* 2, 4 (1996):397–98.

Petrylak, D.P. Metastases suppressers and prostate cancer. *Nature Medicine,* 1, 8 (1995):739–40.

Pietenpol, J.A., and B. Vogelstein. Tumor suppressor genes. No room at the p53 inn. *Nature* 365, 6441 (1993):17–18.

Rubin, E., and J.L. Farber. *Pathology*. Philadelphia: J.B. Lippincott, 1994.

Ruoslahti, E. How cancer spreads. *Scientific American* 275 (1996):42–47.

Weinberg, R.A. The cell cycle clock and cancer. *Scientific American* 275 (1996): 36–37.

_____. How cancer arises. *Scientific American* 275 (1996):32–40.

Wyllie, A.H. Apoptosis. Death gets a brake. *Nature* 369, 6478 (1994):272–73.

CHAPTER 6

Common Adult Cancers

Most lumps and swellings are not cancer. A neoplasm is a new growth, a tumor. Cysts and benign tumors frequently are present as lumps. A common misconception is that all tumors are cancer. In fact, most tumors are harmless bumps that stop growing after a few months or years and do no harm. Rarely, however, even a benign tumor can have catastrophic effects. For example, a benign neoplasm located in a critical area such as the midbrain, by putting pressure on surrounding vital structures, will cause severe neurological problems or even death. Benign tumors of endocrine glands can secrete excess hormones and cause metabolic problems. For example, a cortisol-secreting adrenal adenoma will cause Cushing's syndrome. An insulin-producing adenoma of the pancreas will produce the same effects as an insulin overdose—low blood sugar, collapse and coma. Mostly, however, the clinical significance of benign tumors is that they produce lumps that must be distinguished from cancer.

The detailed medical terminology used to classify cancer confuses the layperson. We classify all cancers histopathologically, by their microscopic appearance. For practical purposes, we can simplify things considerably by omitting pathologic detail. Most cancers arise from the layer of cells known as epithelium that lines the surface of many tissues and organs; these are called carcinomas. So, the common types of adult cancers are lung carcinoma, breast carcinoma, prostate, carcinoma of the skin, carcinoma of the ovary, carcinoma of the colon, and so on.

Table 6.1 lists typical examples of a small number of types of cancer, to illustrate their names, what they look like under the microscope (differentiation), and their typical locations. Most tumor types can occur in almost every location. There are some exceptions, such as gliomas, which occur only in the brain and spinal cord.

We subclassify each cancer by its organization and differentiation. Adenocarcinomas grow with a microscopic pattern resembling glandular structures; this is glandular differentiation. If the glandular differentiation resembles very closely the structure of normal glands, the tumor is well-

Table 6.1 Histopathologic Classification of Cancer

Cancer type	Differentiation	Where it commonly occurs
Adenocarcinoma	Composed of glands	Intestine, lung, uterus, ovaries
Squamous cell carcinoma	Composed of squamous cells and keratin (like normal skin)	Skin, lung, cervix
Ductal carcinoma	Composed of glands (a subtype of adenocarcinoma)	Breast, pancreas
Papillary carcinoma	Composed of microscopic fingerlike structures	Thyroid, ovary, breast
Undifferentiated carcinoma	Composed of round or spindle-shaped cells with no identifiable resemblance to normal tissue	Lung (any organ)
Leiomyosarcoma	Composed of cells resembling smooth muscle cells	Uterus, intestine
Liposarcoma	Composed of immature fat cells	Trunk, limbs
Osteosarcoma	Composed of immature bone cells	Near knee or shoulder joints
Lymphoma	Composed of lymphocytes (immune cells)	Lymph nodes (anywhere)
Leukemia	Composed of bone marrow cells	Bone marrow, blood
Glioma	Composed of glial cells such as astrocytes	Brain, spinal cord

differentiated. If it barely resembles normal glands it is poorly differentiated. If it is somewhere in between these extremes it is intermediately differentiated. If there is no resemblance to any normal tissue, the tumor is undifferentiated. (See figure 6.1.) Well-differentiated cancers only slightly deviate from normal adult mature tissue whereas undifferentiated tumors resemble the primitive rapidly dividing tissue of an early embryo.

At the top left of figure 6.1, oval squamous cells get progressively smaller and flatter as they differentiate. Malignant squamous cells resemble normal cells to varying degrees. As they get progressively more poorly differentiated and undifferentiated they lose all resemblance to normal squamous cells. On the top right, the mucosal lining forms normal glands. Tumors arising from this also form glands and are said to show glandular differentiation. Gland-forming cancers are adenocarcinomas. As they grow more undifferentiated, they no longer have the ability to form glands and

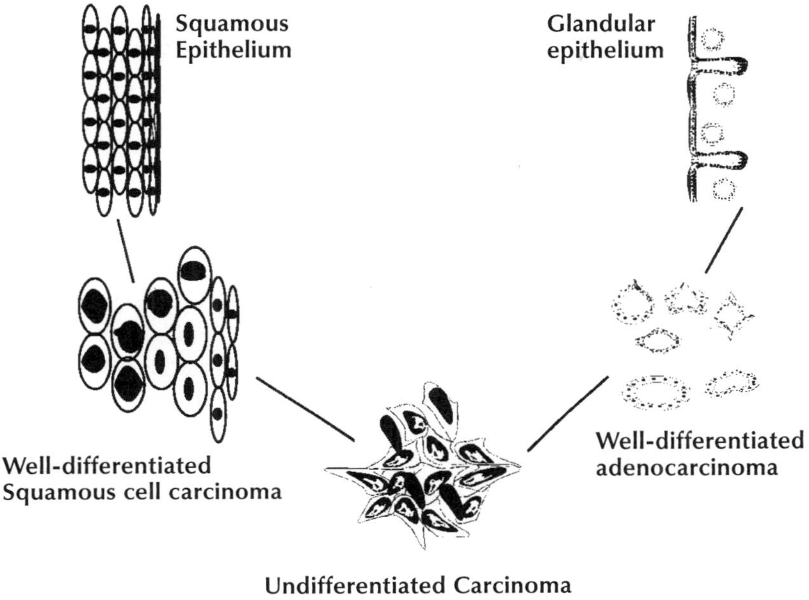

Figure 6.1. Tumor differentiation.

they too become undifferentiated. Differentiation correlates closely with tumor grade and speed of growth. Well-differentiated carcinomas tend to be low-grade and slow-growing. Undifferentiated carcinomas are usually high-grade and grow rapidly.

Finally, the tumor is graded as low, intermediate, or high grade according to how aggressive the tumor cells look under the microscope. The size and shape of the tumor cells, the number of cells filling each microscopic field, the staining intensity of the nuclei (using hematoxylin dye as a nuclear stain), and the number of mitoses present all contribute to the grade.

Grade refers to how abnormal individual tumor cells look under the microscope. It is closely related to differentiation (which relates more to how the cells are organized and resemble normal tissue). In the top left group in figure 6.2., each cell is similar to its neighbor. All the cells are approximately the same size and shape. In particular the nuclei are very similar. In the intermediate-grade tumor, nuclei are larger, darker, and more irregular. In the high-grade tumor, the cells are very irregular in shape and size. In particular, the nuclei show great variability and appear much darker than normal. The nuclear appearance reflects the extensive DNA and chromosomal abnormality in each cell.

Mitosis is the process of nuclear splitting in a cell undergoing division, and the presence of many mitoses usually indicates a rapidly growing tumor. Tumor grade correlates closely with differentiation; low-grade tumors are well differentiated and high-grade tumors are poorly differentiated. The importance of tumor grade and differentiation is that they provide some clues about how we can expect the tumor to behave. Often they also indicate how we might expect a tumor to respond to chemotherapy or radiation therapy. (The concepts of differentiation and grade are relevant to all forms of cancer.)

Malignancies arising in tissues beneath the epithelium and in soft tissue, muscle, and bone constitute the second major group of cancers, the sarcomas. These are far less common than carcinomas. Their histopathological classification depends also on their tissue of origin and their differentiation. A sarcoma arising from muscle in the intestine is a leiomyosarcoma. The *myo* part of the name indicates that it is derived from or differentiating toward muscle cells. The prefix *leio* indicates that the cells are attempting to produce smooth muscle—they show smooth muscle differentiation. If a sarcoma shows skeletal muscle differentiation, it is a rhabdomyosarcoma. *Rhabdo* refers to striated or skeletal muscle. Sarcomas arising from bone-forming cells (osteoblasts) are osteosarcomas. From cartilaginous cells (chondroblasts) we have chondrosarcomas, and so on. Strictly speaking, they are named more accurately on their differentiation patterns than on their tissue of origin. Benign tumors also show muscle and other types of connective-tissue differentiation. The benign counterpart of a leiomyosarcoma is a leiomyoma. This the commonest of all tumors. In the uterus, this benign neoplasm is called a fibroid and it is a common cause of irregular menstrual bleeding.

Leukemias and lymphomas make up the third major category (after carcinomas and sarcomas). These originate from blood and immune cells. There are many subtypes, and like cancers in other tissues some grow slowly and indolently whereas others pursue an explosive and fulminant course.

Some cancers do not fall neatly into any of these categories and often have a separate category for themselves. Rare cancers such as malignant teratomas and carcinosarcomas show combined epithelial and connective-tissue components.

After a pathologist diagnoses a malignant tumor, the following microscopic information is available: (1) the name of the tumor, (2) its differentiation, and (3) its grade. Any or all of these carry important implications for the patient, as they influence the most appropriate treatment and the prognosis. One additional clinical variable, namely, tumor stage, is essential for proper management. Tumor stage defines the extent of tumor spread at the time of diagnosis. There are many staging systems. However, all are

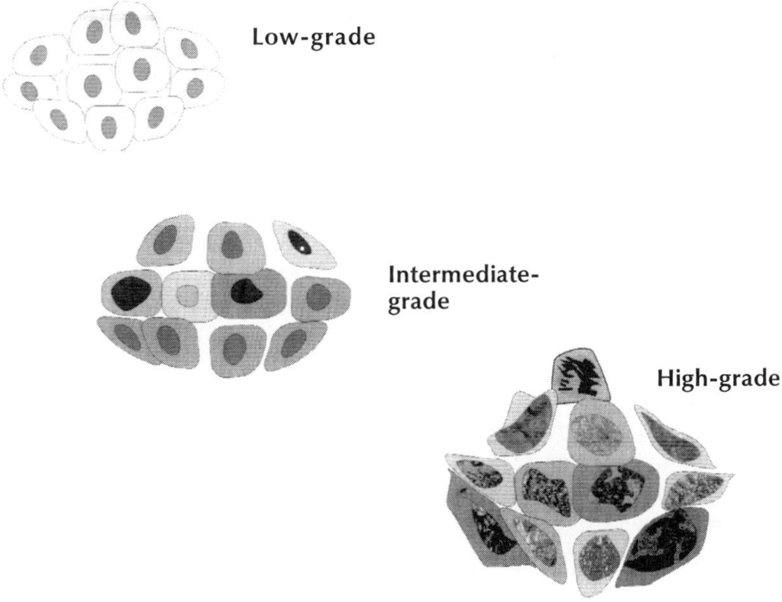

Figure 6.2. Microscopic appearance of tumor grade.

based on the same principle. Each tumor is staged as I, II, or III, according to whether the cancer appears (1) confined to its site of origin, e.g., breast, (2) has spread to adjacent lymph nodes, e.g., in the axilla (armpit), or (3) has spread to distant sites, e.g., lung, liver, or bone. In general, the lower the stage the greater the chance of cure. In contrast, high stage tumors (those that have metastasized) are curable in only a few types of cancer such as testicular cancer, leukemia, and malignant lymphomas. When the surgeon removes the entire tumor and draining lymph nodes, for example in a breast or colon cancer, the pathology report will include an accurate stage. For some cancers, radiological techniques, especially CT scans, provide the stage. Radiological staging takes place before surgery and often determines whether surgery will be beneficial.

Using the earlier analogy to the garden weed, we would expect that removal of the tumor before it had shed its seeds into nearby tissues would guarantee a cure. In practice, it is often impossible to say at the time of diagnosis, with absolute confidence, that a few undetected cells have not metastasized. This means that a number of tumors classified as stage I by currently available techniques will in reality be stage II or III, unbeknownst to the surgeon or oncologist. Furthermore, we do not fully understand yet the clinical relevance of micrometastases. Intuitively, we expect these cells to proliferate, to grow into large tumor metastases, and to kill the patient. We do not know for sure whether they always progress relentlessly, or whether they sometimes regress and are killed by our own defense mechanisms (this last seems most likely). One of the goals of chemotherapy is to eradicate micrometastases that are hidden from our investigation tools. Currently, much effort and research resources are directed at the accurate identification of micrometastases. In some circumstances, their identification may alter treatment and offer patients a better chance of cure.

Lung Cancer

Lung cancer is the number-one cancer killer in men and women, with 177,000 new cancers and 158,700 deaths in the United States in 1996. However, statistics released at the end of 1996 show a new downward trend, attributable to a new awareness of the dangers of smoking and a subsequent reduction in the number of cigarettes smoked.

We have two lungs; each is housed in one side of our chest cavity. Anatomically, they partially surround the organs in the central chest—heart, thymus gland, esophagus (gullet), the great blood vessels entering and leaving the heart (aorta and vena cava), lymph nodes, a variety of nerves, and a small amount of connective tissue. Each lung resembles an inverted tree with its trunk and dividing branches getting smaller and smaller as they reach the periphery and ending in thousands of leaves. We need to modify the analogy to a tree in a few ways. First, its entire inside from its base upward must be hollowed out, leaving only the bark and a thin layer of underlying wood on the outside. It now resembles a series of tubes, of large caliber at the base and decreasing in diameter as they grow outward (peripheral branches). Second, replace the leaves with bunches of berries. Now remove the flesh of each berry, leaving intact the berry skin. This fragile skin can now inflate and deflate like a balloon with each breath of air arriving from the connecting branches. The berries are the lung alveoli, and these are lined by oxygen-absorbing cells. Third, although we have two lungs, we have only one, as it were, tree trunk. This is the trachea, connecting to the outside world through the back of the mouth.

The trachea begins at the opening of the larynx (the voice box). It bifurcates in the midchest region, and its branches are called bronchi. A film of thin, flat, smooth tissue, like wet plastic wrap, surrounds the entire outer surface of the lung and folds onto the inner chest wall and the upper surface of the diaphragm. This lining is the pleura. Rhythmic contractions of chest wall muscles, located between the ribs and muscles in the diaphragm, control the constant inhalation of air. Elastic tissue in the connective tissue of the lungs contracts automatically and expels the air. The diaphragm muscle beneath the lungs forms the boundary between the contents of the chest and the contents of the abdomen. It has a small opening to allow the esophagus and great vessels pass to and from the abdomen.

The outer wall of the trachea, corresponding to the tree bark, is moderately rigid and consists of muscle reinforced by cartilage rings. A specialized type of epithelium (respiratory epithelium) lines the inner surface of the trachea and its branches, the bronchi. The epithelial cells making up this epithelium are tall and rectangular (referred to as columnar cells) and contain thousands of hairlike filaments on their luminal (inner) surface that come in contact with the constantly flowing air. These filaments, called cilia, wave like sea anemones. Their motion is purposeful and always directed upward and outward toward the mouth. The cilia are bathed in a slightly sticky, viscous fluid, and this fluid traps tiny dirt particles and stray bacteria in the incoming air. Once trapped in the bronchial fluid (mucus), the cilia sweep them up into the mouth where they are swallowed unconsciously with saliva and then killed and digested in the stomach by gastric acid and enzymes. If more than a normal amount of fluid comes from the bronchi, e.g., in smokers or in someone with a respiratory infection, the excess fluid is coughed up. The bronchi terminate in the respiratory alveoli (the berries).

Lung cancer arises anywhere and everywhere along the lining of the respiratory tract, from bronchi to alveoli. However, the vast majority of cancers begin in the bronchi nearest the trachea. Here, as the respiratory passage begins to narrow, the bronchial epithelium takes the maximum impact from whatever carcinogens are in the inhaled air—hot smoke, nicotine, various tars, and other chemicals in cigarette smoke (figure 6.3). The greater the number of cigarettes smoked over a lifetime, the greater the insult to the lining epithelium.

Gradually, under repeated irritation, columnar cells change to squamous cells, similar to those lining the mouth. This is an adaptive protective change. Squamous cells resist chemical irritation better than columnar cells. This change from one type of cell to a different cell type is termed metaplasia, and it is reversible. When smokers give up the cigarettes, their bronchial cells return to normal columnar cells. If they continue to smoke, the squamous cells become dysplastic and eventually may become malignant.

Lung cancer is classified pathologically as either squamous-cell carcinoma, small-cell undifferentiated carcinoma, large-cell undifferentiated carcinoma, or adenocarcinoma. This latter group arises from dysplastic columnar cells that have not first changed to squamous cells. The large-cell

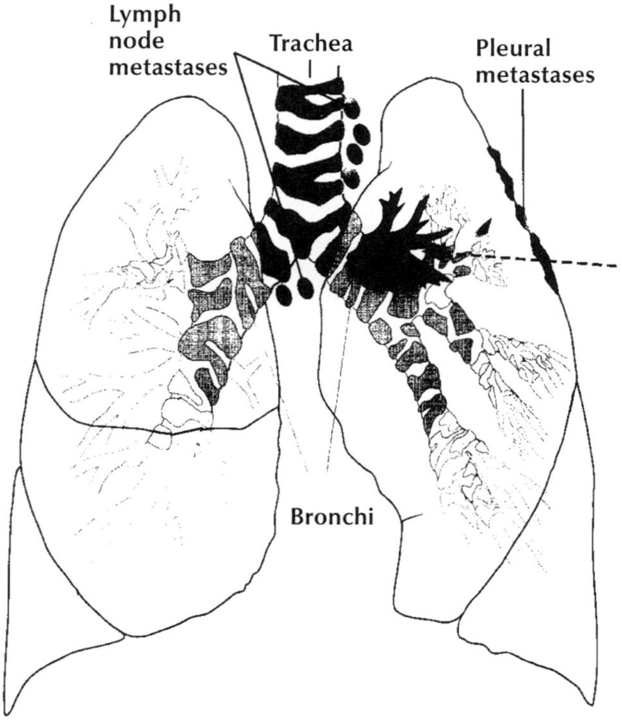

Figure 6.3. Lung cancer, showing pleural invasion and lymph node metastases.

undifferentiated carcinomas include squamous-cell and adenocarcinomas that have lost all evidence of differentiation, thus the term *undifferentiated*. Small-cell undifferentiated carcinomas, also called oat-cell carcinomas (early observers likened the microscopic appearance to oats), are somewhat special and different from the others. They have different biological characteristics that make them extremely aggressive.

Treatment strategy often begins by classifying lung cancer into one of two major groups, small-cell and non-small-cell cancer. In general, the prognosis for most patients with lung cancer is poor. For small-cell carcinomas it is dismal. At the time of diagnosis most lung cancers have spread outside the bronchi and lungs, to lymph nodes, pleural cavity, or distant organs. Only pancreas, esophagus, and liver cancer have poorer survival rates. The overall five-year survival rate for lung cancer is 13 percent. For small-cell carcinoma it is less than 2 percent.

Lung-cancer symptoms are caused by the location and size of the primary tumor or by some complication arising from its spread outside the lung. Symptoms due directly to the tumor include chronic cough or spitting up blood (hemoptysis) or sputum streaked with blood, from ulceration of the tumor surface. If the tumor blocks a major bronchus, the patient may have breathlessness, especially if he or she already has bronchitis and emphysema. A partially blocked bronchus cannot eliminate mucus, which then pools and stagnates beyond the obstruction. In time, the mucus becomes infected and progresses to pneumonia. Furthermore, because of the poor drainage, pneumonia in such a case responds very slowly to antibiotic treatment. Repeated episodes of pneumonia in a middle-aged or elderly patient should alert the family physician to the possibility of lung cancer, especially if the patient is a smoker. Under these circumstances, if nothing appears on a chest X-ray, the patient will often be referred for a bronchoscopy.

Some cancers penetrate the bronchial wall and lung and infiltrate the pleura. This produces a pleural effusion (a collection of fluid in the pleural cavity) that may be large enough to compress and collapse the underlying lung and cause shortness of breath (dyspnea). Involvement of the outer layer of pleura, which lines the inner aspect of the chest wall, often causes discomfort or pain. Infiltration of the recurrent laryngeal nerve, which runs beside one of the bronchi, paralyzes one of the vocal cords and causes hoarseness. Sometimes patients have symptoms outside the chest due to metastatic tumor at some distal site, e.g., bone or brain. Bone metastases cause pain, often in the spine or hip. Sometimes bones with such tumors fracture after minimal or no apparent trauma. Brain metastases might cause headache, epilepsy, or a stroke.

A third group of symptoms, called paraneoplastic syndromes, are due to metabolic abnormalities caused by chemicals discharged by the tumor cells. We know which chemicals are responsible for some of these syndromes. Others are still a mystery. As mentioned above, the small-cell cancers have some unique biological properties. They resemble the primitive cells of an embryo and have some characteristics of neuroendocrine cells, which are the cells that secrete hormones that influence nerve functions. These cells, when examined by the electron microscope, contain tiny packets of chemicals and hormones within membrane-bound granules. These chemicals and hormones are secreted into the bloodstream and produce their effects just as if the patient were taking high-dose medication or hormone injections.

The best-known syndrome caused by small-cell carcinoma is Cushing's syndrome. Tumor cells secret ACTH (adrenocorticotrophic hormone), which stimulates the adrenal gland to produce vast quantities of cortisone and similar hormones. Cushing's syndrome is characterized by (1) obesity, with obvious excess fat deposition in the abdomen, in the upper back (producing a buffalo hump), and in the face (giving it a round, red, moonlike appearance), (2) very thin, fragile skin, (3) hypertension (high blood pressure), and (4) osteoporosis (brittle, thin bones, prone to fracture).

How could cancer of the lung, arising from the lining of the bronchial tree, cause Cushing's syndrome?

In an earlier discussion we saw that all cells contain a full complement of genes, but that some genes switch off during the process of differentiation and are not expressed and remain nonfunctional. They no longer send production messages to the cytoplasmic ribosomes. Under normal circumstances, cells in the pituitary gland at the base of the brain produce a peptide called ACTH (adrenocorticotrophic hormone). This peptide stimulates the adrenal gland to produce cortisone. Lung-cancer cells, growing out of control, reactivate their ACTH-producing genes. The tumor cells behave like pituitary cells out of control and drive the adrenal gland to produce large quantities of corticosteriods. These then cause the Cushing's syndrome. Only a small proportion of lung cancers do this. Other cancers, elsewhere in the body, may also produce ACTH; they produce many other hormones also. Paraneoplastic syndromes sometimes precede the detection of cancer; more often they begin late in the course of the patient's illness. In general, such paraneoplastic syndromes, apart from terminal wasting, are relatively uncommon.

Other syndromes associated with small-cell carcinoma are caused by (1) an imbalance in salt and water metabolism, (2) abnormal calcium metabolism, (3) toxicity to muscles and nerves, and (4) a form of arthritis affecting the wrists and fingers. Weight loss and wasting, similar to that seen in patients with AIDS, is common with terminal cancer. This is due, in part, to poor nutritional intake; more often it is due to a chemical known as TNF (tumor necrosis) factor, secreted by the cancer.

Although small-cell carcinoma is the main culprit, from time to time the other lung cancers (as well as cancers elsewhere in the body) cause paraneoplastic syndromes. Furthermore, we now realize that additional mechanisms, other than hormone release, can cause these syndromes. Sometimes the body, in an attempt to destroy the "foreign" tumor, produces antibodies against the tumor cells. Unfortunately, such antibodies occasionally cross-react with normal cells and tissues and destroy them. Each patient will have some combination of the symptoms described above, but thankfully, no patient will have all these symptoms.

How is lung cancer diagnosed? Once the clinician suspects cancer, a series of investigations follow. After a physical examination comes a chest X-ray. This is followed by examination of sputum (coughed-up mucus or spittle) for malignant cells. The most specific and useful procedures are bronchoscopy and biopsy. The bronchoscopist, usually a specialist respiratory physician or thoracic surgeon, inserts a bronchoscope into the trachea and bronchi. This instrument has a high-quality optical lens, a channel for inserting a biopsy forceps, and a camera or video attachment. The operator can look at the tumor, photograph it, and remove a small fragment with the biopsy forceps. This is then diagnosed, classified, and graded by a pathologist, usually within twenty-four hours. Subsequently, a surgeon and radiologist stage the tumor using CT scans. The combined results of the pathologic diagnosis and the radiologic staging will largely determine whether the patient will benefit from surgery. Other critical variables relevant to the therapeutic decision will include the patient's age and general medical condition. These may have a significant bearing on how well the patient is likely to benefit from or even survive major surgery.

Most patients with small-cell carcinoma have widespread metastases at the time of diagnosis and do not benefit from surgery. There are some exceptions, such as patients with very small tumors located in the lung periphery. Patients with non-small-cell tumor types may benefit from surgery if the tumor appears localized by radiological staging procedures. Surgery is usually recommended as a first-line treatment for these patients. Unfortunately, the pathologist frequently finds that the tumor has spread further (outside the lung) than could be seen by the radiological techniques, or even during surgery. Even the most sophisticated scans cannot identify microscopic tumor deposits. However, if the cancer is genuinely stage I, then therapy may offer five-year survival rates up to 75 percent. This optimistic figure does not apply to small-cell carcinomas.

Radiotherapy often melts tumor bulk and alleviates symptoms. However, it rarely cures tumors that cannot be removed by surgery. Chemotherapy often prolongs survival and improves symptoms and quality of life for patients with small-cell carcinoma.

Breast Cancer

Breast cancer is now the number-two cancer killer in American women, accounting for 46,000 deaths in 1996. Until about 1992, it was in the number-one position. Since then, lung cancer has occupied the number-one slot. The analogy of the hollowed-out tree, growing berries instead of leaves, is also helpful to describe the structure of the female breast. Much of the bulky breast tissue beneath the skin is fat and connective tissue (mostly collagen). Embedded with this is a system of ducts and lobules. Each duct corresponds to the tree trunk and branches, and the lobules are the berries. There are approximately twenty duct-lobule units in each breast and these open into the nipple. While the tree analogy is useful to illustrate this outline structure, the breast is, of course, functionally entirely different. Its mission is to make milk, and its basic microscopic structure reflects this function. The ratio of fat to duct-lobule tissue varies with age. Younger breasts have abundant glandular tissue with relatively little fat. This is why young breasts are firm. As they age, breasts lose their glandular tissue and gain more fat. Histologically, each tubelike duct is surrounded by a thin basement membrane (BM). Sitting on the BM are the duct epithelial cells, which are cube-shaped and line the entire duct system until they meet the lobules (branches of berries). The lobules are milk-forming units, and they are lined by specialized milk-secreting glandular cells known as acinar cells. Although they resemble closely the ductal cells, they have the capacity to respond to pregnancy hormones and secrete milk. Lobules have many specialized contractile cells to help excel milk.

The commonest symptom of breast cancer is a lump. It is important to realize, however, that most breast lumps are not cancer. Fibrocystic change and fibroadenomas are much commoner than cancer. Benign fibrocystic change is the commonest cause of a breast lump. This results from years of waxing and waning of female hormones during the menstrual cycle, and it often appears around menopause. It seems that certain parts of the breast either overrespond or underrespond in a nonuniform fashion to female hormones. Small or large cysts and increased glandular tissue produce a palpable lump. Often the surgeon can diagnose such lesions without biopsy. Using a thin narrow-bore needle, the surgeon aspirates straw-colored clear fluid from a cyst to confirm the benign diagnosis. In younger women, fibroadenomas are the commonest cause of a breast lump. These are well-defined benign tumors that need not be removed. However, for peace of mind, most women opt to have them excised. Older medical textbooks often include the observation that "no lady should have a lump in her breast." Fibroadenomas can be removed easily with no residual breast deformity.

Most breast diseases produce one of three symptoms: a lump, pain, or a nipple discharge. The suspicious breast lump is usually hard and attached to surrounding tissue. As it infiltrates normal tissue, it causes a slight dimpling or puckering of the overlying skin. If it lies close to the front and center of the breast, the nipple may retract slightly. As in almost all cancers, pain is not a symptom unless nerves or adjacent structures, such as the chest wall, are infiltrated; neither of these is common with breast cancer. Most nipple discharges are due to benign lesions. Rarely they are caused by cancer growing along the ducts. Therefore, a discharge cannot be ignored, especially if it is blood-tinged. Rarely, breast cancer presents as a persistent nipple rash. This is Paget's disease of the nipple and is diagnosed by a skin biopsy from the nipple.

Breast cancers arise from the epithelial cells lining the ducts and lobules, mostly from ducts. They are classified as ductal or lobular carcinomas, and they may be in situ or invasive. The top left corner of figure 6.4 shows a breast in cross section, with some of the major ducts shaded; these contain ductal carcinoma in situ (DCIS). Nearby ducts are normal. A cross section of a normal duct shows a lining composed of a single layer of cells. These have a uniform appearance and are surrounded by basement membrane. In the magnified view of the DCIS, tumor cells have filled the duct and are piled irregularly on each other. Tumor cells are much larger than normal cells and their nuclei are irregular. The basement membrane is intact, and these tumor cells cannot yet metastasize. This type of abnormality usually produces no breast lump but can be identified by mammography. Whether they are invasive or not is critical, because only the invasive carcinomas can metastasize and kill the patient. About 85 percent of breast cancers are invasive at the time of diagnosis. Before the era of mammography about 95 percent were invasive at the time of diagnosis; since the 1990s many more breast cancers are diagnosed at the in situ stage. Invasive ductal carcinoma is the commonest type. There are a number of histological subtypes, and most of these have no special significance. However, some do. For example, some tumors are exceptionally well differentiated and composed entirely of small, relatively innocuous glands. These are called tubular carcinomas. Doctors now recognize why this special type is important—it has an excellent prognosis. Although they are invasive, unlike most other invasive breast cancers they rarely metastasize widely. Even those tubular carcinomas that metastasize to lymph nodes usually do not spread any further. Most invasive breast cancers are invasive ductal carcinomas: NOS (not otherwise specified) or NST (no special type). The second major type is invasive lobular carcinoma. This also has a few (although less important) histological subtypes.

Ductal carcinoma in situ (DCIS) is the commoner of the in situ types. It too has several subtypes. Until recently surgeons and other clinicians paid little attention to the subtypes. They treated all types of DCIS in the same way—by simple mastectomy. With changing surgical attitudes, there has been a major switch away from mastectomy to minimal surgery, with conservation of as much breast tissue as possible. We subtype DCIS into high-grade and low-grade DCIS. As you might expect, high-grade DCIS has a greater tendency to recur and become invasive. Usually, the surgeon does not know whether the DCIS is high-grade or low-grade until after surgery and the pathology report arrives. If it is high-grade, the patient will usually receive radiation therapy to the entire breast. This is effective in preventing a recurrence. Some recent studies recommend radiotherapy for all patients with DCIS, irrespective of grade, who have lumpectomies or seg-

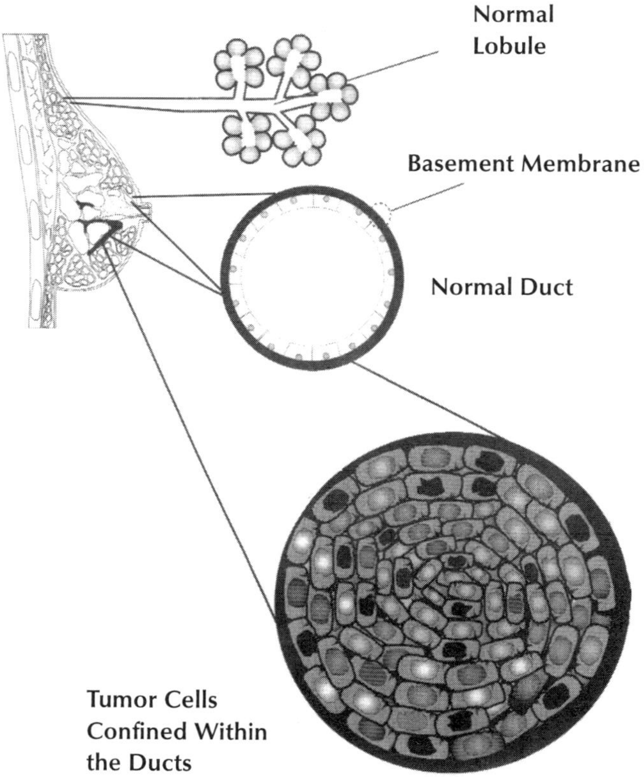

Figure 6.4. Ductal carcinoma in situ (DCIS) of the breast.

mentectomies. The most important points about DCIS are that it often does not need a mastectomy and the cure rate is close to 100 percent.

Lobular carcinoma in situ (LCIS) is a controversial topic from the therapeutic viewpoint. It produces no symptoms or signs, and mammography cannot identify it. During surgery the surgeon can neither see nor feel it. LCIS turns up unexpectedly under the pathologist's microscope as an incidental finding. The surgeon removes some form of lump—a cyst or some other benign lesion—and the pathologist finds LCIS lurking unobtrusively between benign glands and cysts.

We know surprisingly little about the biology and natural progression of LCIS. What we do know is that patients with LCIS are at risk for developing breast cancer sometime in the future. Some studies estimate that

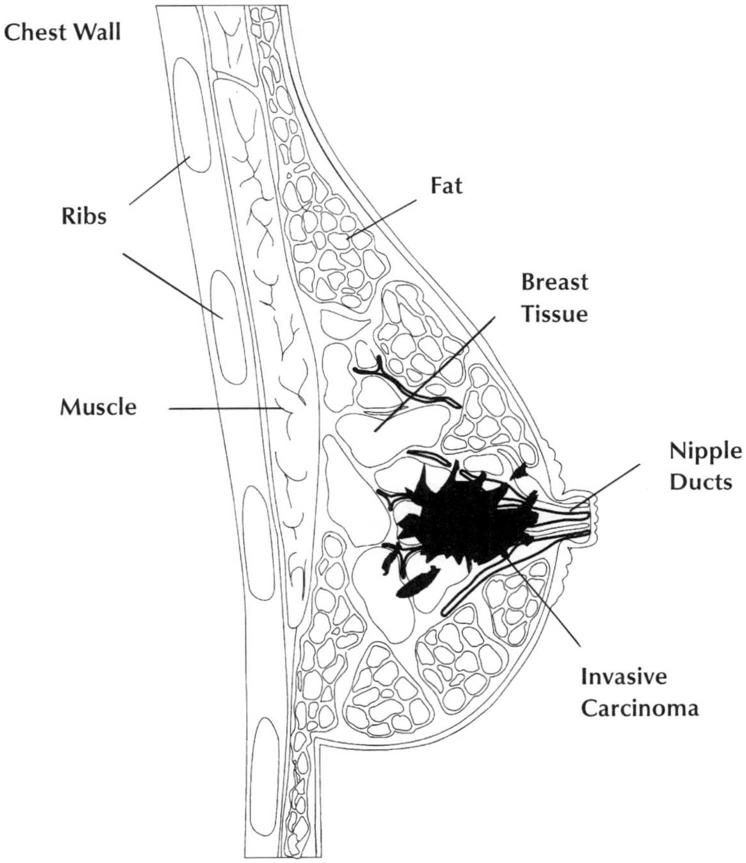

Figure 6.5. Invasive breast cancer.

there is a 25 percent chance of developing cancer within twenty-five years. What we do not know is which part of the breast will get the cancer, or even whether the cancer will arise in the same breast as the original LCIS or in the other one. Many authorities believe that LCIS is not a malignant lesion but rather some form of risk indicator. To add to the confusion, when infiltrating cancer does develop it is more often ductal than lobular. Thirty years ago surgeons overrated the risk, and many women had bilateral mastectomies for what we now know is a slow-growing preneoplastic lesion that usually does not progress to invasive cancer. Nowadays most patients, on their surgeon's advice, adopt a wait-and-see attitude. Usually, surgeons recommend no further therapy for LCIS discovered incidentally. However, some patients still opt for prophylactic mastectomy.

Chapter 13 discusses the topic of mammography and its role in screening for breast cancer. Many surgeons omit mammography if a lump is obviously suspicious and instead decide to get cells or tissue immediately for microscopic diagnosis, either by fine-needle aspiration or by biopsy. Once the diagnosis of cancer is made, it is classified and staged. Grading, based on the microscopic appearance, relies on identifying how well differentiated it is, how abnormal the tumor nuclei appear, and how rapidly it appears to be growing (pathologists estimate this by counting mitoses). The size of the tumor, whether it infiltrates nearby muscle and whether it has spread to axillary lymph nodes, decide the stage.

Some tumors have receptors that bind to the female hormones, estrogen and progesterone, and analysis of these receptors gives useful extra information. The clinician advises on the best treatment taking all these findings into consideration. Additional information is gained by analyzing the tumor receptor status, i.e., whether the tumor cells have hormone receptors. Based on these variables and on the patient's age, menopausal status, and general medical condition, a therapeutic decision is made on whether the patient requires (1) additional surgery, e.g., a mastectomy or removal of more tissue surrounding the tumor margins, reconstructive surgery, or prosthesis implant, (2) radiotherapy, (3) chemotherapy, or (4) antihormone treatment, i.e., the drug Tamoxifen.

It is likely that in the near future therapy will also take into account the results of some newer molecular biology tests, such as analysis of abnormal tumor DNA profiles (ploidy analysis), cell kinetics, and measurement of oncogene activity. The overall prognosis for invasive breast cancer patients has not improved dramatically in the past thirty years. This is because so many patients have distant metastases at the time of diagnosis. Breast cancer, stage I (confined to breast) and II (breast with involved axillary nodes), is curable in a high percentage of patients. If breast cancer can be diagnosed at an early stage, either while it is in situ or minimally invasive, the change of getting a complete cure approaches 100 percent. The goal of breast-screening programs is to identify such curable cancers.

Cancer of the Prostate Gland

The walnut-sized and walnut-shaped prostate gland lies at the base of the urinary bladder (figure 6.6.). Its secretions surround sperm with a variety of chemicals and fluid necessary for normal function. Most men know little or nothing about their prostate gland. It is a hidden internal organ and until relatively recently the public had no idea that prostate cancer was common or that it killed so many men. It is commoner than breast cancer (317,000 new cases in 1996) and kills almost as many men every year (41,400 deaths in 1996). Unlike breast cancer, however, it is uncommon under the age of 50; the median age of prostate cancer patients is 72. A small percentage of prostate cancers are familial. As a man gets older, the likelihood of getting this cancer increases greatly. We know from autopsy studies that more than 50 percent of men who reach the age of 90 have prostate cancer. Many prostate cancers are small, slow-growing, and are not life-threatening. Furthermore, they often have been sitting harmlessly in their prostates for many years. If these cancers had been detected at the age of 65 and removed, their owners would not have gained anything from treatment. Indeed, many would have suffered from postoperative complications, and possibly some would have died. This type of information poses a dilemma for many patients and their doctors.

A small low-grade tumor, found incidentally or by a cancer-screening program, presents the physician and patient with a major therapeutic decision—should it be removed or is it safe to adopt a watch-and-wait policy? As a man gets older, his prostate enlarges slowly. This is so common as to be considered normal. In many men it obstructs the flow of urine from the bladder. This enlargement, benign prostatic hyperplasia, is treated by medication or more commonly by removing the obstructing tissue through an endoscope. The procedure—a transuretral resection—removes slivers of prostatic tissue. This is how an incidental carcinoma is found. Alternatively, a tiny asymptomatic nodule may be found by the patient's physician at a routine checkup or after a blood test shows a slightly raised prostate specific antigen (PSA). More on PSA later.

The prostate gland consists mostly of glandular tissue, much like breast lobules. Glands open into the urethra through a series of short ducts. The urethra is the channel through which urine flows from the bladder to the external surface. In males it also forms the channel for expulsion of semen, intermixed with prostatic fluid.

Most prostatic cancers arise from the glandular tissue. Occasionally they originate from the larger ducts. The neoplastic cells develop from lining epithelial cells. Dysplastic and preinvasive epithelial changes, similar to ductal carcinoma in situ of the breast, precede the onset of cancer. However, those changes are not identified as frequently as in the breast. When they are found, it is difficult to predict their clinical behavior, and therapeutic decisions are not as clear-cut as with DCIS of the breast. Invasive prostatic carcinomas form glands—they are adenocarcinomas, and they may be well or poorly differentiated like other carcinomas. A special grading system, the Gleason grading system, unique to the prostate, reflects the pat-

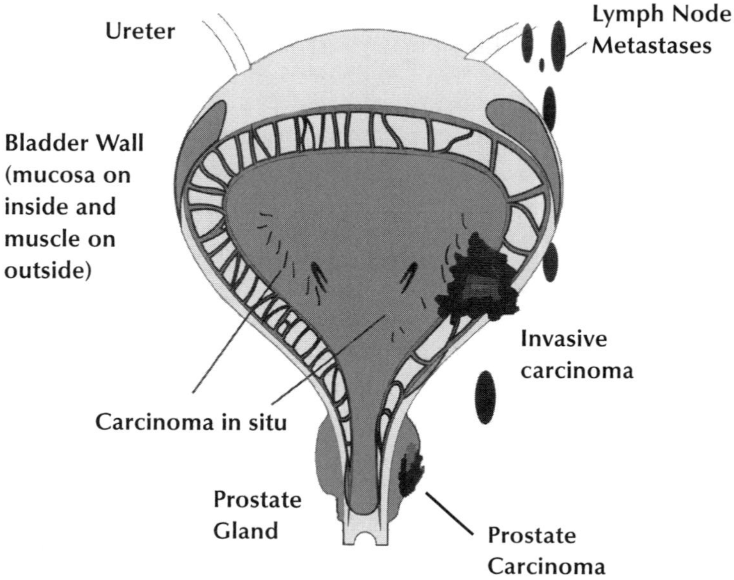

Figure 6.6. Prostate and bladder cancer.

terns of tumor differentiation. The Gleason system is a powerful tool for predicting aggressiveness and metastatic potential.

Staging is critical for therapy and prognosis. Prostate cancer staging is complicated. Tumor stage can be stratified into many substages. However, the basic principles are similar to those used elsewhere, and stage is based on answers to the following questions: Is the tumor confined to the prostate, and if so, is it confined to one lobe of the prostate or not? What size is the tumor? Has the tumor spread locally beyond the prostate, and if so, how far, and are any adjacent structures infiltrated? Has the tumor spread to lymph nodes or to more distant organs? The vertebrae and pelvic bones are the favored sites for prostatic metastases.

Therapeutic options take into consideration the tumor grade and stage and the patient's age and general medical condition. Treatment options include (1) watch and wait for evidence of progression, (2) surgery, (3) radiotherapy, (4) chemotherapy, and (5) hormonal treatment, including castration to remove the major source of androgens. The type and extent of the surgery and radiotherapy depend on the tumor extent and location. Many prostate cancers are partially dependent on male androgens for continued growth. Antiandrogen medication and castration are often very successful in relieving pain from spinal metastases.

The overall five-year survival rate is 85 percent and for small localized cancers it exceeds 95 percent. Patients with distant metastases have a five-year survival of less than 30 percent.

The Gastrointestinal Tract

The gastrointestinal tract consists of esophagus, stomach, small intestine, and large intestine: cancer can arise anywhere, in any tissue. Mostly, however, it arises from the epithelium lining the surface—the part closest to the lumen and in contact with food. The basic structure of the intestine is similar throughout its length. It is a hollow tube composed of three layers: epithelium, muscle, and serosa. The cells lining the inner epithelial layer of the stomach secrete acid. In the stomach and in the small intestine the epithelial cells also secrete digestive enzymes. In addition, epithelial cells in the small intestine absorb digested food; this is their main function. In the large intestine their main function is to absorb water. The muscle layer propels food and its residual leftovers along 30 feet (9 meters) of intestinal tract from mouth to anus. Unlike the muscles in your arms and legs, you have no voluntary control over this muscle; appropriately it is called involuntary muscle. The physical presence of food and a battery of chemical signals instruct this muscle to contract in a series of coordinated waves known as peristalsis.

The serosa is a flimsy, slippery, thin membrane that envelopes the intestine and separates it from other abdominal organs. It is similar to the pleura surrounding the lung. If it is damaged or absent, loops of intestine tend to stick to each other, preventing the normal flow of its contents. Throughout the intestine there are some variations in this basic structure. The mucosal lining of the esophagus is composed of squamous epithelium, identical to that lining the mouth, and it is very similar also to the outer layer of the skin. The esophagus moves food from mouth to stomach, where digestion beings. The squamous lining protects it against rough, partially chewed food particles.

The stomach is not a mere hollow tube like the rest of the intestine; it resembles a small bag with an entrance tube (the esophagus) and an exit tube (the small intestine). Food churns about and remains for a few hours in the stomach before peristalsis moves it forward into the small intestine. A final variation is a test-tube-like outpouching from the first part of the large intestine. This is the appendix, which in humans appears to have no useful function except possibly to give employment to surgeons.

Cancer of the Esophagus

Cancer of the esophagus resembles cancer of the skin, lung, and cervix; pathologically it is a squamous cell carcinoma. Figure 6.7 shows the lower part of the esophagus and the center of the stomach with separate cancers. Both cancers have been put in the same picture for illustration only. It would be very rare for a patient to have a carcinoma of the esophagus and cancer of the stomach at the same time. Each tumor has spread through the wall and has metastasized to lymph nodes. The esophageal cancer has arisen from squamous epithelium and is a squamous carcinoma. The stomach cancer has arisen from glandular epithelium and shows glandular differentiation. It is an adenocarcinoma. Elsewhere in the intestine, cancers are gland-forming and are classified as adenocarcinomas. Cancers in the lower portion of the esophagus sometimes arise in glandular mucosa resembling the mucosa in the stomach or intestine; these are also adenocarcinomas.

This situation whereby normal esophageal squamous epithelium is replaced by glandular tissue is called intestinal metaplasia. An esophagus partially lined by glandular tissue is termed a Barrett's esophagus, and it is premalignant. Chronic acid regurgitating from the stomach into the lower esophagus, over one or two decades, transforms the squamous mucosa to glandular mucosa. In some patients, this constant acid irritation causes dysplastic changes, followed by cancer.

Apart from Barrett's esophagus, a couple of preexisting abnormalities such as achalasia and congenital mucosal webs appear to be risk factors. Achalasia is a disorder of the lower esophagus caused by failure of its distal segment (that is, its stomach end) to relax properly during swallowing. The esophagus with achalasia has poor motility and is widely dilated above the diseased segment. Food with its possible carcinogens remains lodged and in contact with the mucosa for hours or days before passing into the stomach. A number of statistical associations have identified possible relevant causative factors or cofactors. High alcohol consumption and cigarette smoking are risk factors. Nitrosamine, a chemical present in some foods, is another possible culprit.

Irrespective of its pathology, cancer of the esophagus produces the same symptoms. The patient complains of difficulty in swallowing (dysphagia) and a sensation of discomfort and food sticking somewhere behind his or her breastbone (the sternum). At first this unpleasant sensation is mild. As the tumor grows and obstructs the passage of food, the condition gradually gets worse. There are also many benign causes of dysphagia. To identify the obstruction as cancer, the doctor passes an endoscope into the esophagus and biopsies the tumor.

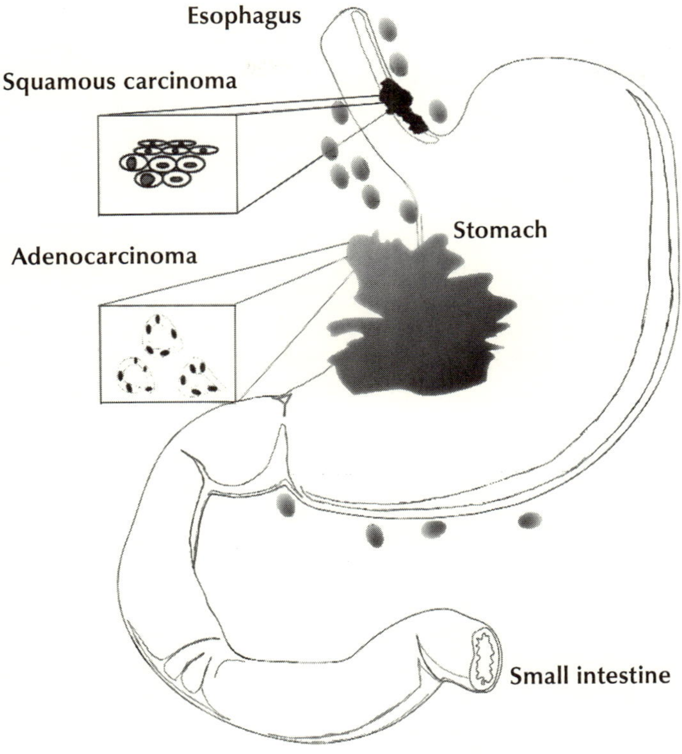

Figure 6.7. Cancer of the esophagus and stomach.

Therapy depends on location and stage of the tumor and the patient's general condition. Most esophageal cancers are advanced at the time of diagnosis and the prognosis is poor, with a five-year survival rate of less than 5 percent.

Cancer of the Stomach

Stomach cancer arises from the mucosa; it is an adenocarcinoma. (See figure 6.7.) The incidence of stomach cancer is falling through the western world, possibly because of changes in our diets and eating habits. The incidence remains high in certain countries, such as Japan. There it is seven or eight times more common than in the United States. Like most cancers, its cause is unknown. Longstanding peptic ulceration, pernicious anemia, and certain dietary factors such as nitrosamines are known risk factors. A tiny spiral bacterium, *Helicobacter pylori*, has captured the imagination of epidemiologists as a possible causative agent for some gastric cancers. This organism causes chronic gastritis, and some researchers think it may also cause cancer—not just carcinoma (an epithelial malignancy), but also a rarer and less serious form of gastric cancer known as gastric lymphoma. Presently, we have insufficient evidence to know for sure if this bacterium is carcinogenic.

Patients with gastric cancer often have vague symptoms. Some patients complain of just poor appetite. Others have loss of energy or weight loss. Others have some type of upper abdominal discomfort or pain. Sometimes the pain is similar to that of a peptic ulcer. In many patients, bleeding from the surface of the cancer produces anemia. Sometimes, a gastric cancer is diagnosed at an early stage, while it is still in situ or minimally invasive. More often, it is advanced, i.e., it has spread beyond the stomach at the time of diagnosis, and in these patients the prognosis is very poor.

Cancer of the Small Intestine

Curiously, cancer of the small intestine is rare. For decades doctors have wondered why. The small intestine is called small because its diameter is small, not because it is short. In fact, it is more than 20 feet in length, and much longer than any other part of the intestine. Statistically, one might expect a greater number of cancers in this organ. Yet this is not so. Furthermore, the type of cancer arising in the small intestine is commonly malignant lymphoma, cancer of the immune cells, the lymphocytes. The usual explanation offered for the rarity of small intestinal cancer is that food carcinogens pass rapidly through this segment of intestine, where they are diluted by a large quantity of intestinal fluid and juices. The contact time between carcinogens and any one part of the small intestine is short. This is unlike the situation in the stomach and large intestine (colon), where contact time is long. Furthermore, the colon absorbs fluid and concentrates fecal contents and any carcinogens that they might contain.

Like cancer in other parts of the intestine, small intestinal cancer may bleed from its surface and cause anemia. Because the contents of the small intestine are fluid, the lumen of the gut may not become obstructed until tumor growth fills the lumen. When this happens, it causes severe pain and vomiting. Before this, it may cause mild pain by interfering with normal peristalsis.

Cancer of the Colon and Rectum

The contents of the first part of the large intestine (colon) are similar to those in the small intestine; they are fluid. Gradually, as these contents make their way toward the end of the colon, water is absorbed and the feces become solid. The rectum, just inside the anus, is the final part of the gastrointestinal tract, and feces remain here until expelled. In figure 6.8, just above the rectum, a large carcinoma has infiltrated through the bowel wall and has spread to lymph nodes and liver. This is classified as a Dukes stage D carcinoma. The box in the lower right shows the microscopic appearance of the tumor. Tumor cells are arranged around central spaces, i.e., they are forming glands. This is an adenocarcinoma.

Colon cancer, striking 150,000 Americans each year, is the second commonest cancer, after lung cancer. In the United States it kills 55,000 each year. About 5 to 10 percent of colonic cancers are hereditary. Most of them are due to recently discovered mutations in a few genes, on chromosomes 2 and 3. These genes are named MSH2 and MLH1, and their function is to repair damaged DNA. Mutated genes fail to protect colonic mucosa from carcinogens and lead to hereditary nonpolyposis colon cancer (HNPCC). Other hereditary colon cancers are much rarer and grow on a background of hereditary polyps. The best-known and most thoroughly studied polyposis syndrome is familial adenomatosis polyposis (FAP). In FAP the rogue gene, on chromosome 5, is transmitted from either mother or father to all their children, who develop thousands of colonic polyps during childhood and adolescence. These polyps, if they are not removed by colectomy, invariably progress to cancer. Frequently, multiple polyps become malignant simultaneously.

Other risk factors for colon cancer are longstanding ulcerative colitis and spontaneous (nonhereditary) polyps. Ulcerative colitis is a chronic inflammatory disease affecting the colonic mucosa. The cause is unknown, and its severity ranges from mild to disabling. In some patients it affects only the distal colon (near the rectum) and rectum. In other patients it involves the entire colon. Those patients who have longstanding (more than ten years) inflammation of the entire colon are most at risk. Older studies indicated that the risk was about ten times as great as for the normal population; more recent studies suggest that the risk is considerably less than this.

As we get older, our colons have a propensity to grow polyps. Thirty percent or more of the western population over the age of 50, have one or more colonic polyps, and a tiny proportion (about 1 percent) become malignant. These are small glandular growths (adenomas), of varying size, that protrude into the colon. Although they can occur elsewhere in the intestine, they are rare outside the colon. The risk of malignancy is proportional to their size and histopathological structure. Those less than 2 cm in diameter have little risk: those greater than 4 cm are especially at risk. The histopathological features that increases the risk for malignancy are severe

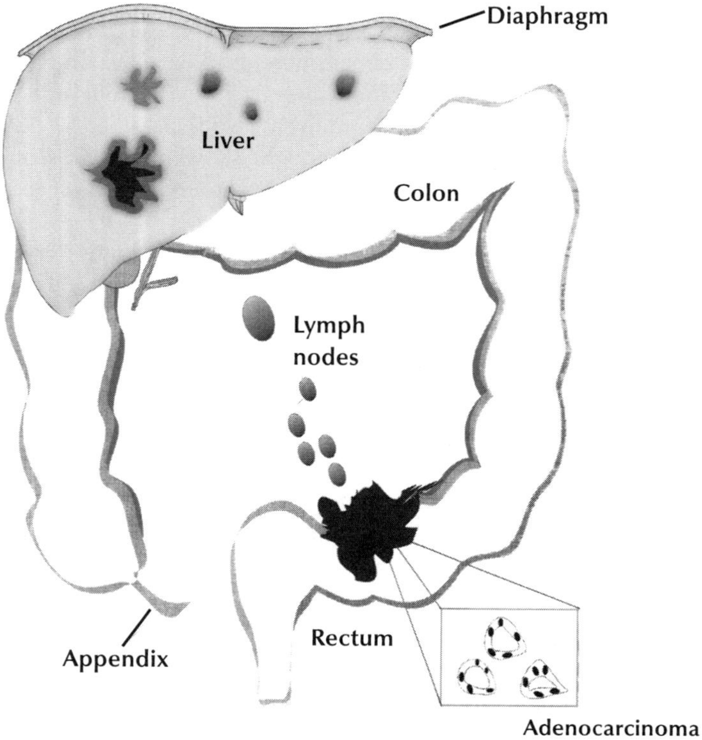

Figure 6.8. Colorectal cancer.

dysplasia and a villous structure; villous tumors have fingerlike projections (*villi*) growing from the surface.

Polyps with a pure villous structure are classified as villous adenomas; those with a pure glandular structure are tubular adenomas. Those with mixed tubular and villous components are tubulovillous adenomas. The greater the size and the greater the villous component, the greater the cancer risk. While only a small proportion of polyps become malignant, almost all colonic cancers arise from polyps. Theoretically then, if we could eliminate all polyps we could prevent colon cancer. This is the rationale behind colon screening programs.

Colonic polyps grow silently and asymptomatically. They sometimes bleed a little from their surface, and if this is sufficient to cause anemia they may reveal themselves during a workup for anemia. If they are located in the rectum and bleed sufficiently, the patient, to his or her alarm, may notice blood on the surface of the feces. Sometimes polyps are found during the course of a workup for some unrelated intestinal symptoms. Since they are premalignant, the usual practice is to remove them by snaring them through a loop on the colonoscope. If they are very large, open abdominal surgery may be necessary. In keeping with what one might expect for premalignant lesions, they begin to appear about ten years before colonic cancers develop. Stated another way, statistics show that patients with colonic polyps are about ten years younger than those with colon cancer.

Anatomically, the large intestine consists of ascending, transverse, descending, sigmoid, and rectal segments. The ascending (proximal) colon is situated in the right side of the abdomen; its first part is called the cecum. The transverse segment runs from right to left across the top of the abdomen, just beneath the diaphragm; the descending, sigmoid, and rectal (distal) segments are located in the left side of the abdomen and in the pelvis. These seeming anatomical trivia in fact have some relevance to the patient with colon cancer, and to the surgeon (as discussed in the paragraph below on treatment).

As we saw earlier, the prevalent hypothesis suggests that something in the feces (coming from our food) converts normal epithelial lining cells into neoplastic cells. Because fecal carcinogens are more concentrated and spend greater time in contact with the mucosa of the left side of the colon, we would expect the greatest incidence of polyps and cancers in this region. So it is. Polyps and cancers are far commoner in the rectum and last part of the colon than they are in the first part. Furthermore, left-sided colon cancers tend to produce different symptoms and have a better prognosis than right-sided cancers. Small, early cancers of the cecum and ascending colon produce no symptoms, apart from anemia due to blood loss. Blood leaked into the lumen of the ascending colon mixes with liquid feces and may not be seen by the patient; liquid feces bypass the growing tumor, unobstructed. By the time the cancer produces symptoms, such as vague abdominal pain or altered bowel habit, it is often large, has infiltrated through the bowel wall, and has metastasized. In contrast, left-sided cancer is in contact with solid feces, and any narrowing of the lumen tends to produce symptoms related to minor degrees of obstruction. Small, early cancers can interfere with fecal movement, producing altered bowel habit (alternating constipation and diarrhea or blood-stained feces. The irritated bowel mucosa sometimes secretes excess mucus mixed with feces and the patient may notice the abnormality.

Almost all colorectal cancers are adenocarcinomas. Dukes staging is the most widely used staging system for colon cancer. Tumors confined to the mucosa and submucosa are called Dukes A; those involving the outer muscle layer are Dukes B; those involving lymph nodes draining the colon are Dukes C; those cancers that have spread to the liver are Dukes D. Veins normally drain from the colon to the liver, and blood-borne metastases go to the liver before metastasizing to other organs. The five-year survival for Dukes A is nearly 100 percent, for Dukes B it is 60 to 80 percent, for Dukes C 35 percent, and for Dukes D less than 1 percent. A number of recent trials suggest that surgery might improve survival for a small number of selected patients with Dukes D tumors.

The first and often the only treatment is surgery. The type of surgery required to treat left- and right-sided colon cancers is different. The surgeon's task in either case is to remove the entire tumor with a rim of uninvolved colon and surrounding abdominal tissue and to suture the normal remaining colonic segments so that the continuity of the lumen remains intact. The arterial blood supply is different in different parts of the colon, and the arterial distribution dictates how much colon must be removed. In practice this means that for right-sided tumors the entire right colon must be removed, whereas for left-sided tumors only a small segment of colon requires excision. Fortunately for the patient, the end result is the same—a normal, functional colon. However, a tumor located in the low rectum, just above the anus, does not have a segment of normal colon between it and the anus, and it is often necessary to remove the anus with the tumor. This destroys the anal muscle sphincter and would leave the patient with fecal incontinence if treated the same way as more proximal tumors. To get over this problem, the surgeon designs a new opening for the proximal colon in the abdominal wall—a colostomy. Feces are collected in a special colostomy bag. With time and training, the patient learns to accept this. Surgeons can sometimes excise a low rectal tumor without destruction of the anal sphincter, if it is a small early cancer.

Malignant Lymphoma

Malignant lymphoma is classified into two main groups, Hodgkin's disease and non-Hodgkin's lymphomas (NHL). Over the past fifteen years scientists and molecular biologists have greatly enhanced our knowledge and understanding of the non-Hodgkin's lymphomas. In many ways, we know more about these lymphomas at the molecular level than we do about any other cancer. However, Hodgkin's disease and its neoplastic cells remain a mystery. Despite extensive research, we still do not know the cell of origin of Hodgkin's disease and its cause is completely unknown. Paradoxically, despite our lack of understanding, the treatment of Hodgkin's disease is far more successful than treatment for the non-Hodgkin's lymphomas. Hodgkin's disease is very sensitive to chemotherapy and radiation therapy.

Hodgkin's Disease

One of the main oncology success stories over the past twenty-five years has been the improved treatment of Hodgkin's disease. Before the new era of medical and radiation oncology, this cancer was invariably fatal. Now, therapy cures most Hodgkin's patients. Nevertheless, there are still 7,500 new cases and 1,500 deaths every year in the United States The microscopic appearance of Hodgkin's disease is characteristic, and pathologists classify it into four subtypes: (1) lymphocyte-predominant, (2) nodular sclerosis, (3) mixed cellularity, and (4) lymphocyte-depleted. In the past this classification was critical, as it predicted which patients would survive for years and which patients would not. The lymphocyte-predominant variety had the best prognosis and the lymphocyte-depleted the worst. Although it is still used, this classification is no longer of such critical importance, since chemotherapy is effective against all subtypes. CT scans and bone marrow biopsy determine the tumor stage. In common with general principles relating to all cancers, low stage (early) Hodgkin's is easier to cure than advanced disease. With most cancers, advanced stage is almost never curable. However, many patients with advanced Hodgkin's are cured, and modern therapy cures almost all stage 1 patients.

Patients with Hodgkin's disease usually complain of painless lymph node enlargement. Large lymph nodes appear as swellings or glands in the neck, armpits, or groin region. Sometimes they arise at multiple sites simultaneously. Some patients also have intermittent fever, night sweats, or weight loss. These are commonly called B symptoms (there are no "A" symptoms). X-rays or CT scans identify involved lymph nodes deep within the body, in the chest or abdomen. Histopathological examination of an excised node establishes the diagnosis. Localized disease responds well to radiotherapy, and this may be the treatment choice for some patients with stage 1 disease and no B symptoms. Chemotherapy has the advantage of acting systemically, and it destroys small tumor deposits that might have escaped detection during the staging procedures. Oncologists frequently use chemotherapy as standard firstline treatment and use additional radiotherapy to eradicate bulky tumor masses (often in the chest). If a relapse occurs after initial radiation treatment, chemotherapy is still effective and usually successful.

Non-Hodgkin's Lymphoma

Non-Hodgkin's lymphoma refers to a group of malignancies arising from the immune cells (lymphocytes). This group is considerably larger than Hodgkin's disease, with 52,700 new cases in 1996 and 23,300 deaths.

Like the immune cells from which they arise, they can be classified as B cell or T cell lymphomas. This is their immunological classification, and it has some relevance to prognosis, in that T cell lymphomas tend to be somewhat more aggressive. However, standard histopathological classification gives more useful prognostic information, and in general, the type of chemotherapy used will depend on the microscopic appearance of the cancerous cells.

If you look up a detailed classification of lymphomas in a medical textbook, you are guaranteed to come away confused; there are dozens of types. However, as with most cancers, it is possible to simplify them by reducing the classification to three grades, low, intermediate, and high. Grade is determined by the size of the tumor lymphocytes and whether their growth pattern resembles the normal follicles in a lymph node or not.

Some molecular changes help to distinguish lymphoma from other conditions that occasionally mimic lymphomas. These molecular markers can also help find micrometastases in staging procedures such as bone marrow biopsies.

Like Hodgkin's disease, non-Hodgkin's lymphoma usually presents with enlarged lymph nodes. However, it often begins with involvement of other organs, such as the salivary gland (in the jaw), stomach, or small intestine. These are called extranodal lymphomas. Often the patient has fever or other B symptoms. These lymphomas are frequently disseminated widely at the time of diagnosis; bone marrow involvement is common. Treatment varies from intense chemotherapy and bone-marrow transplantation to no treatment at all, depending on the tumor classification, stage, age of the patient, and the patient's general medical condition. An example of the "no treatment group" would be a 72-year-old man with no symptoms other than a lump in the side of his neck. A surgeon removes this lump and the pathologist reports that it is a lymph node replaced by low-grade lymphoma. There is no evidence of disease elsewhere. The next question is how the patient should be treated. The doctor tells the patient and his family that for his type of lymphoma treatment will not prolong his life. To treat this patient makes no sense. If the disease recurs locally or the patient develops symptoms at a later date, some therapy may then be of value.

Although the overall survival for low-grade lymphomas is better than for high-grade lymphoma, there is one notable exception and paradox. Some rapidly proliferating high-grade lymphomas are very sensitive to chemotherapeutic drugs and total cure is often possible. In contrast, low-grade lymphomas are indolent and slowly progressive, and although long-term survival is common, complete cure is rare. These tumor cells often grow at a slower rate than normal cells and are resistant to chemotherapy. They accumulate in the body and continue to grow because they lack cell-eliminating genes; they escape normal apoptosis. Leukemias are similar to lymphomas in many ways. They often arise from the same B and T lymphocytes and there are low-grade and high-grade leukemias. The main difference from lymphoma is that they begin with widespread involvement of the bone marrow and also involve the circulating blood. When lymphoma involves the marrow it does so at a later stage.

Leukemia

Leukemias are cancers of the bone marrow and peripheral (circulating) blood cells. The center diagram of figure 6.9 shows bony trabecula with the entire marrow space occupied by tumor cells. The higher magnification in the lower diagram shows that the normal marrow cells have been replaced by lymphoblasts. Similar cells flood the peripheral blood and travel to other tissues.

The structure and function of marrow is described briefly in chapter 7, in the childhood leukemia section. In adults, the variety of leukemias is far greater than in children. The pathological classification is complicated. However, we can simplify it by grouping many of the subvarieties under two major headings and just a few subheadings. First, we classify them as either acute or chronic. Then we subclassify them by their cell of origin. The acute leukemias are acute lymphoblastic and acute myeloid (or myeloblastic); the cells of origin are either lymphocytes or granulocytes (also called myeloid cells). These leukemias have a rapid onset (thus the name acute). Leukemia cells infiltrate and destroy the normal marrow cells. As a result, patients are anemic and bleed easily into their skin, mouth, and other tissues. They are susceptible to severe infections, often by microorganisms that are harmless for people with a normal immune system.

Cancer cells in acute leukemias are immature or poorly differentiated and are called blasts, either lymphoblasts or myeloblasts. Many biological variables affect how they respond to treatment. For example, acute lymphoblastic leukemia in children has a far better prognosis than the same disease in adults. New immunological and molecular biology markers also help identify different prognostic groups.

The chronic leukemias are rarely found in children. They increase in frequency during middle and old age. As their name suggests, they have a slow onset. There are two major types, chronic lymphocytic leukemia (CLL) and chronic myeloid leukemia (CML). Patients with chronic lymphocytic leukemia present with generalized lymph node enlargement—in the neck, armpit, and groin regions. Lymph nodes inside the body cavities and the

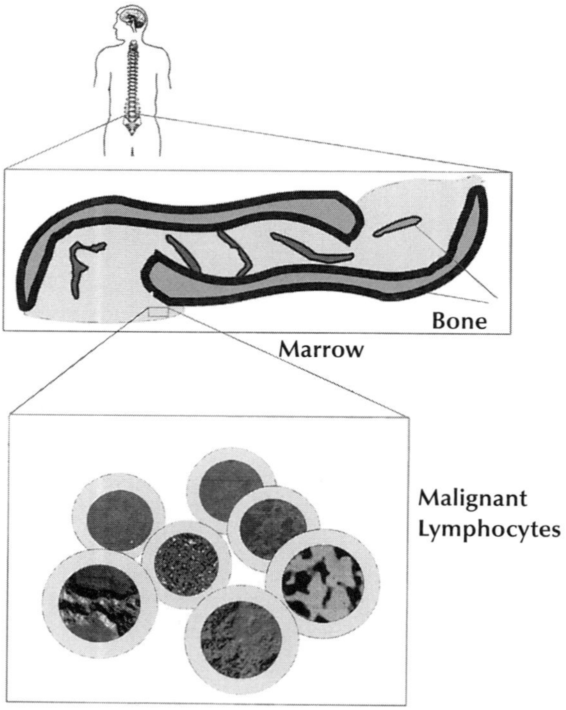

Figure 6.9. Acute lymphoblastic leukemia.

spleen are also enlarged. The bone marrow and peripheral blood are overrun by small, mature, well-differentiated lymphocytes. These grow and accumulate slowly like the low-grade lymphoma cells. In fact, in many ways they are very similar to lymphoma cells. The major difference between them is their clinical presentation. Chronic lymphocytic leukemia arises in the bone marrow and spills into the peripheral blood. It involves lymph nodes later. Low-grade lymphomas are based primarily in lymph nodes and infiltrate the bone marrow at a later stage; often the peripheral blood is not involved. Like low-grade lymphoma cells, CLL cells accumulate slowly, have poor apoptosis control, and are relatively resistant to chemotherapy.

Chronic myeloid leukemia (CML) has a slow onset but enters an accelerated growth phase after a few years and then transforms into acute leukemia. Myelocytes (granulocytes) at different stages of maturation replace the bone marrow and involve the peripheral blood. They also infiltrate and enlarge the spleen to such a degree that it causes abdominal discomfort or pain. Chronic myeloid leukemia cells have a characteristic chromosomal abnormality—the Philadelphia chromosome. This is a useful diagnostic marker. Until recently, CML was invariably fatal and CML patients had a much shorter survival than those with CLL. The terminal blast transformation resisted all forms of therapy. Now, many patients with CML are cured by bone marrow transplantation.

The treatment for all forms of leukemia and lymphoma is chemotherapy, with one notable exception. Patients with low-grade lymphoma or chronic lymphocytic leukemia are often elderly and asymptomatic. These patients usually do not benefit from chemotherapy. Symptoms are treated as they arise. For example, slowly progressive anemia may need blood transfusions or infections may need prompt and rigorous antibiotic treatment.

The statistics for the entire group of leukemias show that in 1996 (in the United States) there were 27,600 new cases and 21,000 deaths. The next chapter, on childhood cancer, contains additional information on leukemia.

Myeloma

In addition to the leukemias, there is one other common type of bone-marrow malignancy—multiple myeloma. This is cancer of the plasma cells. These cells are derived from B lymphocytes, and their job is to manufacture and secrete antibodies. Like other lymphocytes, they play an essential role in the immunological policing of all tissues. They specialize in fighting infections. When myeloma strikes, these cells form cancerous nodules throughout the bone marrow that destroy their surrounding bony cage. Bone destruction causes osteoporosis, microfractures, and pain, usually in the spine (vertebral column). As the nodules replace the bone marrow, the patient develops anemia. They continue to secrete immunoglobulins, but these proteins are functionless and useless for fighting infections. The abnormal immunoglobulins appear in the blood and urine and their detection aids in diagnosis.

Myeloma is a disease primarily of the elderly, although it also afflicts the middle-aged. In 1996 there were 14,400 new cases and an estimated 10,400 deaths. It is slowly progressive and relentless. Radiation therapy helps to alleviate back pain. Some drugs produce a partial remission and alleviate symptoms. Cure is exceptionally rare, and the overall objective of treatment is to control and reduce plasma cell proliferation and to keep the patient as comfortable as possible.

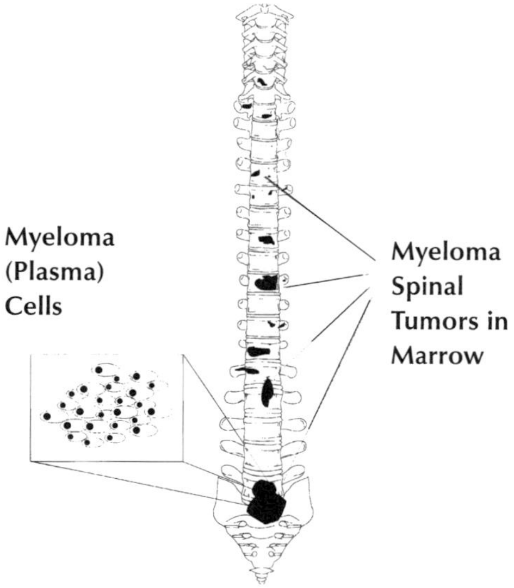

Figure 6.10. Multiple myeloma.

Cancer of the Ovary

The (two) ovaries are shaped like almonds, but twice as large (figure 6.11). They lie within the pelvis and connect to the womb by the fallopian tubes. The ovary's job is to send a ripe ovum (egg), ready for fertilization, into the womb each month. This assignment begins in early puberty and finishes at menopause. Each ovary consists of a mixture of hormone-producing cells called "sex-cord stroma," ova and their precursor cells called "germ cells," and a specialized surface epithelium. Each cell type breeds a different type of cancer. Numerically, the epithelial cancers are overwhelmingly more common than the others. Each year more than 26,000 American women get ovarian cancer, and it kills 14,000. We have very little understanding of what causes it. A small percentage of ovarian cancers are due to hereditary mutations. Because it is located deep in the pelvis, it produces no symptoms until it is large enough to cause abdominal discomfort or swelling. Sometimes patients have irregular menstrual cycles. Once the diagnosis is suspected, an ultrasound examination of the pelvis confirms the presence of an ovarian tumor and may show features suspicious for malignancy.

During surgery, the gynecologist notes very carefully whether the

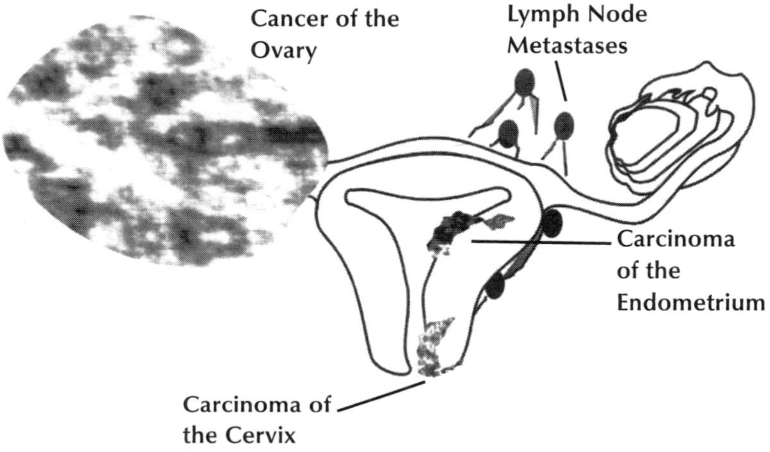

Figure 6.11. *Cancer of the ovary, uterine cervix, and endometrium.*

tumor has penetrated the capsule on the surface of the tumor and whether it has spread anywhere else in the abdomen. This information is critical for proper staging and influences the subsequent decision about whether chemotherapy is necessary.

Often, ovarian cancer is bilateral, and usually the patient is postmenopausal. The obvious surgery for such patients is to remove both ovaries and the uterus. Pathological examination verifies the extent of tumor invasion and spread. Unlike most other cancers, preoperative biopsy is not generally recommended. Proper pathological evaluation requires examination of the entire tumor, after surgical removal.

When ovarian cancer metastasizes, it spreads to the lining of the abdomen (the peritoneum). There it induces a large accumulation of fluid, known as ascites. This produces abdominal swelling and distension. Later, metastases spread to the liver and other organs. The prognosis depends primarily on the tumor stage at the time of diagnosis. The overall prognosis for ovarian cancer patients is poor, with a five-year survival of only 35 percent. This is because most cancers are at an advanced stage at the time of diagnosis. Patients with stage 1 cancer (confined to the ovary) have an excellent prognosis, with a five-year survival of 90 percent or greater.

In addition to surgery, the choice to apply radiation therapy or chemotherapy depends on each patient's circumstances. Some tumors produce a tumor protein called CA-125 and secrete it into the bloodstream, where it can be detected and measured. It is a useful tumor marker for monitoring the tumor's response to treatment and for detecting tumor recurrence.

Germ-cell cancers of the ovary are uncommon. They occur in younger patients, often in their twenties, and are exquisitely sensitive to chemotherapy. The prognosis for these patients is excellent. The same tumors are commoner in males, where they occur in the testes and have an equally excellent prognosis.

Bladder Cancer

The urinary bladder resembles a soccer ball with three holes (figure 6.6). Two of these connect to the kidneys by the ureters, and they receive a constant trickle of urine, every second of every day. When the bladder is full, its owner gets slightly uncomfortable and empties it through the third opening. The bladder sits within the pelvis, behind the lower part of the abdominal wall, and acts as a reservoir for urine. It is lined by a delicate layer of epithelium, known as transitional epithelium. Muscle surrounds and envelopes the mucosa and is responsible for the expulsion of urine. Throughout a lifetime, the transitional epithelium exposes itself to every waste chemical eliminated by the body. The main function of the kidneys is to purify the bloodstream and to get rid of its waste products by dumping them into the bladder. Here they sit around for hours waiting for the bladder to empty itself. In some ways, it is remarkable that the incidence of bladder cancer is not much higher than its 52,900 annual figure. It kills more than 11,000 Americans each year.

In the past, dye industry workers commonly got bladder cancer. Some of the dye breakdown products were carcinogens. This industrial hazard has now been eliminated. Inhabitants of North Africa, where infestation by the parasite *Shistosoma* is common, have a higher incidence of bladder cancer associated with this infection. In the western world, the most widely known association with bladder cancer is cigarette smoking. Cigarette smoke contains many tars and carcinogens. These are toxic not only to the lung mucosa in direct contact with the smoke but also to those other tissues subsequently exposed to absorbed chemicals. Experts estimate that smoking contributes to 30 to 40 percent of all bladder cancers. There is a clear dose-response relationship; the more you smoke the more likely you are to get bladder cancer.

Bladder cancers and their precursor abnormalities remain silent and asymptomatic for years. Often the appearance of a little blood in the urine is the first symptom. Sometimes patients may have some discomfort and have a sensation of needing to pass urine too often. This is called urinary frequency.

A surgeon or urologist makes the diagnosis by examining the bladder

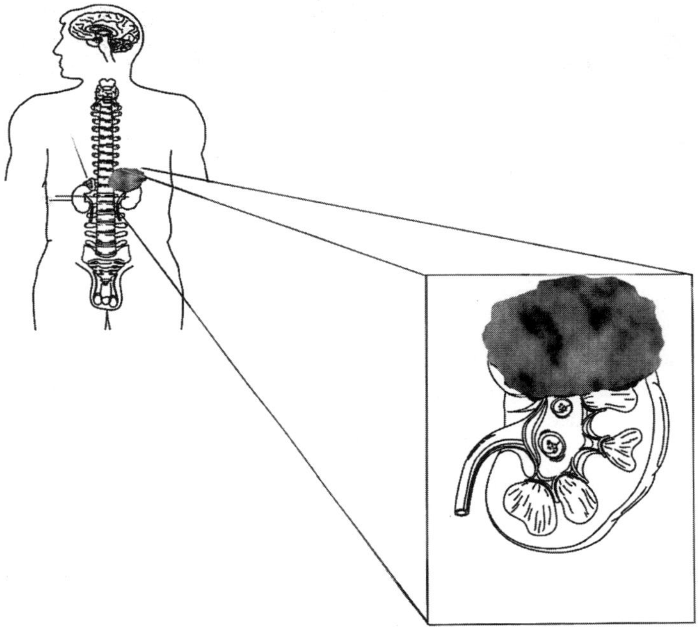

Figure 6.12. Renal cell carcinoma.

mucosa with a cystoscope and by biopsying any abnormal areas. A cystoscope is a special type of endoscope for examining the inside of the bladder. Microscopic examination confirms the diagnosis and provides the grade and stage. Pathologically, most bladder cancers are transitional-cell carcinomas. These are graded as low, intermediate, and high. They are staged according to how deeply they invade the muscle component and whether they have metastasized locally or distally. If the patient has bladder surgery, the stage may have to be revised after the entire bladder and draining lymph nodes are examined. However, most patients require very limited surgery, which is carried out through the endoscope. Superficial (noninvasive or minimally invasive) cancers respond well to this type of surgery. Although these cancers recur frequently, close surgical supervision with repeated cystoscopy produces excellent results. Those patients with deeply invasive tumors often require radical surgery. Some also require radiation therapy. Chemotherapy is valuable as a palliative treatment for some patients. Sometimes chemotherapy is valuable before surgery to reduce tumor bulk, for this makes surgical dissection easier.

Paradoxically, carcinoma in situ of the bladder is often high-grade. Frequently, it involves extensive areas of mucosa, making cystoscopic surgery inadequate. These patients require radical cystectomy. If the malignant cells are confirmed to the mucosa, this type of surgery guarantees cure. The overall five-year survival rate is 80 percent. For very early cancers, it approaches 100 percent. Even those cancers that are not very early, but still localized at the time of diagnosis, have a 92 percent five-year survival rate. Patients with distal metastases at the time of diagnosis have a 6 percent five-year survival rate.

Cancer of the Kidney

The two kidneys sit high up in the back of the abdomen. They are the body's main waste disposal units. Every minute they filter 1.2 liters of blood and continuously clear minute quantities of toxic chemicals from the bloodstream. They also ensure that the body maintains a proper fluid balance.

Two main cancers arise in the kidney. One of these, Wilms' tumor, affects children and is discussed in the next chapter on childhood cancers. The adult form arises from the epithelial cells and is called renal cell carcinoma. It is diagnosed in more than 30,000 Americans, and it kills 12,000, each year. Most kidney cancers are situated on the upper (as illustrated here) or lower pole of the kidney. In adults, cancer of the kidney is a type of adenocarcinoma. In children, it is Wilms' tumor. It commonly metastasizes to lymph nodes, lungs, and bones.

The cause of renal cancer is unknown. Most may be caused by environmental carcinogens. As in bladder cancer, there is a definite link with cigarette smoking. A small number are due to hereditary genetic DNA mutations of the VHL gene (VHL is short for von Hippel-Lindau). Patients with VHL syndrome get familial renal cancer and benign vascular tumors (hemangioblastomas) in the brain and eye. Recently, molecular biologists identified the VHL gene. Even nonfamilial kidney cancers show mutations in this gene. Alterations in the VHL and a number of other newly discovered genes now appear to play a major role in the initiation and progression of kidney cancer.

Symptoms vary from patient to patient. Some complain of blood-stained urine or back pain. Others have weight loss, general malaise, or fever. Some kidney tumors produce no symptoms and are diagnosed by abdominal ultrasound examination that is being performed for some unrelated reason. Surgical excision is the best treatment, and at surgery the tumor-bearing kidney and surrounding soft tissues are removed. Chemotherapy and radiotherapy are of benefit to very few patients.

Although it has a reputation for being unpredictable, most studies show that prognosis depends largely on the tumor grade and tumor stage, just as for most other cancers. The overall five-year survival rate is approximately 55 percent. Patients with localized disease at the time of diagnosis have a five-year survival rate of 87 percent. For those with distant metastases, it is 10 percent.

Table 6.2 shows the incidence and mortality statistics for new cases and deaths in 1996 for other common cancers not discussed in this chapter.

Table 6.2. Annual New Cases and Deaths of Various Cancers in the United States (1996)

	Estimated New Cases	Estimated Deaths
Melanoma (skin)	38,300	7,300
Uterus other than cervix	34,000	6,000
Oral cavity and pharynx	29,490	8,260
Pancreas	26,300	27,800
Brain	17,900	13,300
Cervix	15,700	4,900
Thyroid	15,600	1,210
Larynx (voice box)	11,600	4,250
Testis	7,400	3,700

In addition to the melanomas, basal-cell and squamous-cell carcinomas of the skin account for more than 800,000 cases annually. However, these are rarely fatal.

Bibliography

General

Abeloff, M.A., J.O. Armitage, A.S. Lichter, and J.E. Niederhuber, eds. *American Cancer Society Textbook of Clinical Oncology*, 2d ed. American Cancer Society, 1995.

Buckman, R. *What you really need to know about cancer.* London: Macmillan, 1996.

Cotran, R.S., V. Kumar, S.L. Robbins. *Robbins pathologic basis of disease.* Philadelphia: Saunders, 1994.

De Vita, V.T. Jr., S. Hellman, and S.A. Rosenberg, eds. *Cancer: Principles and Practice of Oncology*, 5th ed. Philadelphia: J.B. Lippincott, 1993.

Grossgebaner, K. The "cancell" theory of carcinogens: Re-evolution of an ancient, holistic, neoplastic, unicellular concept of cancer. *Medical hypotheses* 45 (1995) 545–55.

Orth, D.N. Cushing's syndrome. *New England Journal of Medicine* 333 (1995): 791–803.

Rubin, E. and J.L. Farber. *Pathology*. Philadelphia: J.B. Lippincott, 1994.

Breast

Bellamy, C.O., C. McDonald, D.M. Salter, U. Chetty, and T.J. Anderson. Noninvasive ductal carcinoma of the breast: The relevance of histologic categorization. *Human Pathology* 24, 1 (1993):16–23.

Berg, J.W., and R.V. Hutter. Breast cancer. *Cancer* 75, (1 suppl.) (1995):257–69.

Cady, B. New diagnostic, staging, and therapeutic aspects of early breast cancer. *Cancer* 65 (1990):634–47.

Donegan, W.L. Recent trends in the management of breast cancer. 1. Carcinoma in situ of the breast. *Canadian Journal of Surgery* 35 (1992):361–65.

Eberlein, T.J. Current management of carcinoma of the breast. *Annals of Surgery* 220, 2 (1994):121–36.

Fisher, B. Lumpectomy versus quadrantectomy for breast conservation: A critical appraisal. *European Journal of Cancer* 31A, 10 (1995):1567–69.

Fisher, B., J. Costantino, C. Redmond, E. Fisher, R. Margolese, N. Dimitrov, N. Wolmark, D.L. Wickerman, M. Deutsch, L. Ore, et al. Lumpectomy compared with lumpectomy and radiation therapy for the treatment of intraductal breast cancer. *New England Journal of Medicine* 328 (1993):1581–86.

Foulkes, W.D. and S.A. Narod. Hereditary breast and ovarian cancer: Epidemiology, genetics, screening and predictive testing. *Clinical and Investigative Medicine* 18, 6 (1995): 473–83.

Garfinkel, L., C.C. Boring, and C.W. Heath, Jr. Changing trends. An overview of breast cancer incidence and mortality. *Cancer* 74, (1 suppl.) (1994):222–27.

Maranto, G. Should women in their 40s have mammograms? *Scientific American* 275 (1996):79.

Sainsbury, J.R., T.J. Anderson, D.A. Morgan, and J.M. Dixon. ABC of breast diseases. Breast cancer. *BMJ.* 309, 6962 (1994):1150–53.

Schnitt, S.J., W. Silen, N.L. Sadowsky, J.L. Connolly, and J.R. Harris. Ductal carcinoma in situ (intraductal carcinoma) of the breast. *New England Journal of Medicine* 318 (1988):898–903.

Simpson, J.F., and D.L. Page. Status of breast cancer prognostication based on histopathologic data *American Journal of Clinical Pathology* 102, (4 suppl. 1) (1994): S3–8. [published erratum appears in *American Journal of Clinical Pathology* 103, 1 (1995):115.]

Watson, J.D., J.R. Sainsbury, and J.M. Dixon. ABC of breast diseases. Breast reconstruction after surgery. *British Medical Journal.* 310, 6972 (1995):117–21. [published erratum appears in *BMJ* 310, 6975 (1995):311]

Prostate

Adami, H.O., J.A. Baron, and K.J. Rothman. Ethics of a prostate cancer screening trial. *Lancet* 343, 8903 (1994):958–60.

Brawer, M.K. How to use prostate-specific antigen in the early detection or screening for prostatic carcinoma. *CA: A Cancer Journal for Clinicians* 45, 3 (1995): 148–64.

Coffey, D.S. Prostate cancer. An overview of an increasing dilemma. *Cancer* 71, (suppl.) (1993):880–86.

Epstein, J.I., P.C. Walsh, and C.B. Brendler. Radical prostatectomy for impalpable prostate cancer: The Johns Hopkins experience with tumors found on

transurethral resection (stages T1A and T1B) and on needle biopsy (state TIC). *Journal of Urology* (1994):1721–29.
Garnick, M.B. Prostate cancer: Screening, diagnosis, and management. *Annals of Internal Medicine* 118, 10 (1993):804–18.
Garnick, M.B., and W.R. Fair. Prostate cancer: Emerging concepts, part 1. *Annals of Internal Medicine* 125, 2 (1996):118–25.
Garnick, M.B., and W.R. Fair. Prostate cancer: Emerging Concepts, part 2. *Annals of Internal Medicine* 125, 3 (1996):205–12.
Grove, A. Taking on prostate cancer. *Fortune* 113 (May 13, 1996):32–40.
Handley, M.R., and M.E. Stuart. The use of prostate specific antigen for prostate cancer screening: A managed care perspective. *Journal of Urology,* part 2, 152, 5 (1994):1689–92.
Jaroff, L. The man's cancer. *Time,* 1 Apr. 1996, p. 58.
Kaye, K.W. Prostate cancer: Enthusiasm for screening. *Medical Journal of Australia* 162, 10 (1995): 540–41.
Korda, M. *Man to Man. Surviving prostate cancer.* New York: Random House, 1996.
Pearson, J.D., and H.B. Carter. Natural history of changes in prostate specific antigen in early stage prostate cancer. *Journal of Urology* 152, (5, part 2) (1994): 1743–48.
Roach, M., C. Marquez, H.S. Yuo, P. Narayan, L. Coleman, U.O. Nseyo, Z. Navvab, and P.R. Carroll. Predicting the risk of lymph node involvement using the pre-treatment prostate specific antigen and Gleason score in men with clinically localized prostate cancer. *International Journal of Radiation Oncology, Biology, Physics* 28, 1 (1994): 33–37.
Slawin, K.M., M. Ohori, O. Dillioglugil, and P.T. Scardino. Screening for prostate cancer: An analysis of the early experience. *CA. A Cancer Journal for Clinicians* 45 3 (1995): 134–147.
Stamey, T.A., P.E. Ekman, M.A. Blankenstein, E.H. Cooper, M. Kontturi, H. Lilja, J.E. Oesterling, U.H. Stenman, and A. Turkes. Tumor markers. *Scandanian Journal of Urology and Nephrology. Supplementatum* 162 (1994):73–87.
Takayama, T.K., and P.H. Lange. Radiation therapy for local recurrence of prostate cancer after radical prostatectomy. *Urologic Clinics of North America* 21, 4 (1994): 687–700.
Walsh, P.C. Prostate cancer kills: Strategy to reduce deaths. *Urology* 44, 4 (1994): 463–66.

Lung

Ihde, D.C. Small cell lung cancer. State-of-the-art therapy 1994. *Chest* 107, (6, suppl.) (1995):243S–245S.
Kanters, S.D., J.W. Lammers, and E.E. Voest. Molecular and biological factors in the prognosis of non-small cell lung cancer. *European Respiratory Journal* 8, 8 (1995):1389–97.
Lippman, S.M., S.E. Benner, and W.K. Hong. Chemoprevention. Strategies for the control of cancer. *Cancer* 72, (3, suppl.) (1993):984–90.
Muers, M.F., and R.A. Howard. Management of lung cancer. *Thorax* 51, 6 (1996): 557–60.
Petersen, G.M. Epidemiology, screening, and prevention of lung cancer. *Current Opinion in Oncology* 6, 2 (1994):156–61.

Sarna, L. Lung cancer: The overlooked women's health priority. *Cancer Practice* 3, 1 (1995):13–18.

Strauss, G.M., D.J. Kwiatkowski, D.H. Harpole, T.J. Lynch, A.T. Skarin, and D.J. Sugarbaker. Molecular and pathologic markers in stage I non-small-cell carcinoma of the lung. *Journal of Clinical Oncology*. 13, 5 (1995):1265–79.

Ovary

Barker, G.H. Recent advances in the treatment of carcinoma of the ovary. *British Journal of Obstetrics and Gynecology* 100, 9 (1993):803–5.

Cannistra, S.A. Cancer of the ovary. *New England Journal of Medicine* 329, 21 (1993): 1550–59.

Cannon Albright, L.A., and M.H. Skolnick. The genetics of familial breast cancer. *Seminars in Oncology* 23, (1, suppl. 2) (1996):1–5.

Carlson, K.J., S.J. Skates, and D.E. Singer. Screening for ovarian cancer. *Annals of Internal Medicine* 121, 2 (1994):124–32.

Minelli, L. Ovarian cysts. *European Journal of Obstetrics, Gynecology, and Reproductive Biology*, 65, 1 (1996):81–89.

Montazeri, A., J. McEwen, and C.R. Gillis. Quality of life in patients with ovarian cancer: Current state of research. *Support. Care Cancer* 4, 3 (1996):169–79.

Qazi, F., and W.P. McGuire. The treatment of epithelial ovarian cancer. *CA: A Cancer Journal for Clinicians* 45, 2 (1995):88–101.

Teneriello, M.G., and R.C. Park. Early detection of ovarian cancer. *CA: A Cancer Journal for Clinicians* 45, 2 (1995):71–87.

Tortolero Luna, G., and M.F. Mitchell. The epidemiology of ovarian cancer. *Journal of Cellular Biochemistry Supplement* 23 (1995):200–207.

Melanoma

Elwood, J.M. Screening for melanoma and options for its evaluation. *Journal of Medical Screening* 1, 1 (1994):22–38.

Evans, G.R., and P.N. Manson. Review and current perspectives of cutaneous malignant melanoma. *Journal of the American College of Surgeons* 178, 5 (1994):523–40.

Garland, C.F., F.C. Garland, and E.D. Gorham. Rising trends in melanoma. An hypothesis concerning sunscreen effectiveness. *Annals of Epidemiology* 3, 1 (1993):103–10.

NIH consensus conference. Diagnosis and treatment of early melanoma. *Journal of the American Medical Association* 268, 10 (1992):1314–19.

Colon and Rectum

Bernstein, C.N., F. Shanahan, and W.M. Weinstein. Are we telling patients the truth about surveillance colonoscopy in ulcerative colitis? *Lancet* 343, 8889 (1994):71–74.

Bond, J.H. Polyp guideline: Diagnosis, treatment, and surveillance for patients with nonfamilial colorectal polyps. *Annals of Internal Medicine* 119, 8 (1993):836–43.

Collins, R.H. Jr., M. Feldman, J.S. Fordtran. Colon cancer, dysplasia, and surveillance in patients with ulcerative colitis. A critical review. *New England Journal of Medicine* 316 (1987):1654–58.

Fielding, L.P., and N. Pettigrew. College of American Pathologists Conference XXVI on clinical relevance of prognostic markers in solid tumors. Report of the Colorectal Cancer Working Group. *Archives of Pathology and Laboratory Medicine* 119, 12 (1995): 1115–21.

Macrae, F.A. Screening for colorectal cancer, 1996. *Medical Journal of Australia* 165, 2 (1996):102–5.

Thomas, G. Advances in the genetics and molecular biology of colorectal tumors. *Current Opinion in Oncology* 6, 4 (1994):406–12.

Toribara, N.W. Colorectal cancer. A new look at an old problem. *Western Journal of Medicine* 161, 5 (1994):487–94.

Esophagus and Stomach

Coia, L.R., and E.R. Sauter. Esophageal cancer. *Current Problems in Cancer* 18, 4 (1994): 189–247.

Eidt, S., and M. Stolte. The significance of Helicobacter pylori in relation to gastric cancer and lymphoma. *European Journal of Gastroenterology and Hepatology* 7(4) (1995 Apr.):318–21.

Fennerty, M.B., R.E. Sampliner, and H.S. Garewal. Review article: Barrett's esophagus—Cancer risk, biology and therapeutic management. *Alimentary Pharmacology and Therapeutics* 7, 4 (1993):339–45.

Fuchs, C.S., and R.J. Mayer. *New England Journal of Medicine* Gastric carcinoma. 333, 1 (1995):32–41.

Harrison, J.D., and J.W. Fielding. Prognostic factors for gastric cancer influencing clinical practice. *World Journal of Surgery* 19, 4 (1995):496–500.

Harvey, J.C., and E.J. Beattie. Carcinoma of the esophagus: An overview. *Comprehensive Therapy* 20, 1 (1994):55–60.

Hendlisz, A., and H. Bleiberg. Diagnosis and treatment of gastric cancer. *Drugs* 49, 5 (1995):711–20.

Kirby, T.J., and T.W. Rice. The epidemiology of esophageal carcinoma. The changing face of a disease. *Chest Surgery Clinics of North America* 4, 2 (1994):217–25.

Le Prise, E.A., B.C. Meunier, P.L. Étienne, V.C. Julienne, D.M. Gedouin, J.L. Raoul, M. Ben Hassel, J.P. Campion, and B. Launois. Sequential chemotherapy and radiotherapy for patients with squamous cell carcinoma of the esophagus. *Cancer* 75, 2 (1995):430–34.

Peters, F.T., and J.H. Kleibeuker. Barrett's oesophagus and carcinoma. Recent insights into its development and possible prevention. *Scandinavian Journal of Gastroenterology Supplement* 200 (1993):59–64.

Philip, P.A., and J.A. Ajani. Has combined modality therapy improved the outlook in carcinoma of the esophagus? *Oncology* 8, 9 (1994):37–42.

Recht, A. The role of radiation therapy in treating patients with potentially respectable carcinoma of the esophagus. *Chest* 107, 6 (suppl.) (1995):233S–240S.

Shimizu, S., M. Tada, and K. Kawai. Early gastric cancer: Its surveillance and natural course. *Endoscopy* 27, 1 (1995):27–31.

Simanowski, U.A., F. Stickel, H. Maier, U. Gartner, and H.K. Seitz. Effect of alcohol on gastrointestinal cell regeneration as a possible mechanism in alcohol-associated carcinogensis. *Alcohol* 12, 2 (1995):111–15.

Spechler, S.J. Barrett's esophagus. *Gastroenterologist* 2, 4 (1994):273–84.

Streitz, J.M., Jr., F.H. Ellis, Jr., S.P. Gibb, and G.M. Heatley. Achalasia and squamous cell carcinoma of the esophagus: Analysis of 241 patients. *Annals of Thoracic Surgery* 59, 6 (1995):1604–09.

Viswanathan, V., and D. Fleischer. Esophageal cancer: Diagnosis and treatment. *Gastroenterologist* 3, 1 (1995):3–13.

Woodward, T.A., and B. Levin. Cancers of the stomach and the duodenum. *Gastroenterologist* 3, 1 (1995):14–19.

Small Intestine

Bauer, R.L., M.L. Palmer, A.M. Bauer, H.R. Nava, and H.O. Douglass, Jr. Adenocarcinoma of the small intestine: 21-year review of diagnosis, treatment, and prognosis. *Annals of Surgical Oncology* 1, 3 (1994):183–88.

Lambert, P., A. Minghini, W. Pincus, P. Kolm, and R.R. Perry. Treatment and prognosis of primary malignant small bowel tumors. *American Surgeon* 62, 9 (1996): 709–15.

CHAPTER 7

Childhood Cancer

Childhood cancer differs from adult cancer in many ways, although there are also many similarities. What they have in common is uncontrolled growth, the capacity to invade and destroy normal tissues, and the ability to disseminate widely throughout the body.

Cancer in children is relatively uncommon, afflicting about 1 in every 350 children (younger than the age of nineteen). In the United States there are 10,000 deaths from childhood cancer each year, in comparison to 500,000 adult deaths. However, its incidence appears to be increasing, and it is the disease that most commonly kills from the age of one through adolescence. The common adult cancers—lung, breast, prostate, and colorectal—do not afflict children. The common childhood cancers are leukemia, lymphoma, and cancers of the brain, kidney, bone, and adrenal gland. The leukemias and lymphomas are for the most part similar to adult leukemias, with a few exceptions. However, those pediatric cancers involving the brain, kidney, bone, and adrenal gland are very different from their adult counterparts.

Genetics and environment are partners in causing all cancers. With adult cancers most authorities believe a lifetime of exposure to environment carcinogens is the important factor. Probably fewer than 10 percent of childhood cancers are due to heritable predisposition. Nevertheless, preexisting DNA abnormalities are more important in childhood than in adult cancers. Bad genes are entirely responsible, for example, in special forms of retinoblastoma, Wilms' tumors, and leukemia.

Childhood cancers are caused by genetic alterations. This is not the same as saying that they are hereditary. Many nonhereditary conditions could damage a child's DNA, including environmental agents. The genetic mechanisms underlying hereditary cancers are discussed in chapter 8.

A tiny number of cancers are present at birth. These are congenital cancers that begin during fetal development and manifest themselves within the first few days or weeks of life. The concept of cancer being initiated in a fetus, while still in the presumed safety of the mother's womb, is called prenatal carcinogenesis. More than thirty published epidemiologic studies have looked at the possible prenatal carcinogenic affects of diet, air quality, and other aspects of the mother's environment. Only diethylstilbestrol and possibly prenatal radiation have been connected with prenatal carcinogenesis in any study. Diethylstilbestrol taken by a mother during pregnancy causes a rare cancer that affects adolescent girls and young adults —adenocarcinoma of the vagina. In the 1940s doctors commonly prescribed this drug to prevent miscarriage. Its carcinogenic effects remained unknown for more than two decades. A wide variety of drugs (and radiation) cause defects (teratogenesis) in human embryos. One concept proposed in 1875 was that tiny teratogenic collections of cells that arise during embryonic development might lie dormant for years and then transform into malignant growths (cancer). For the most part, this hypothesis is dismissed nowadays. However, it may have relevance to one childhood cancer in particular. It appears that in infants persisting islands of immature kidney tissue, called nephrogenic rests or nodular renal blastema, predispose the child to the development of Wilms' tumor, which is one of the commonest childhood cancers. Of possible relevance is the interesting fact that there is a greater risk of Wilms' tumor in children with a group of congenital malformations called the Beckwith-Wiedemann syndrome. Although not well documented, it is possible that persistent abnormal fetal tissue might contribute also to some other childhood cancers.

Could something in the father's environment damage his sperm and subsequently cause cancer in his children? This attractive hypothesis tried to explain the occasional "clustering" of childhood leukemias in the neighborhoods of nuclear reactor plants. Again, however, studies have failed to confirm this hypothesis. Similar studies have failed to link cancer with fathers who work in autorepair, welding, television and radio repairs, or in environments with concentrations of electromagnetic fields, paint, hydrocarbons, nitro compounds, exhaust fumes, or insecticides. There are still raging controversies over some environmental conditions, such as electromagnetic waves and cigarette smoke; no doubt studies will continue on the effects of some of these agents. In experimental animals a variety of chemicals induce malformations if given very early in the embryo's development, and cancer if given during later development.

Could prenatal viral infection cause childhood cancer? A few viruses are likely candidates. The human T-cell lymphotrophic viruses (HTLVs) are retroviruses and one of these, HTLV1, is thought to cause a particularly virulent form of leukemia in Japan and the Caribbean area. HTLV1 passes from mother to child, often through breast milk. Some perinatally infected children may subsequently develop T-cell leukemia. There is also some evidence that perinatally acquired hepatitis B and C may cause liver cancer in adults.

The Chernobyl disaster in 1986 has caused a superabundance of radiation-induced thyroid cancers in children. Likewise we know that therapeutic radiation given to many children and young adults in the 1950s caused thyroid cancer many years later. The expected increase in leukemias after Chernobyl, however, has not yet appeared.

Despite claims that high-tension cables and their electromagnetic waves might cause cancer in children, there is insufficient evidence to confirm such claims.

Leukemia

Leukemia is the commonest childhood cancer and it differs from the adult form in that it is almost always of the acute variety. The chronic leukemias seen in adults almost never affect children.

Normal bone is made up of an outer core of thick bone called the cortex, to give it strength, and an inner mazelike meshwork called the medulla. Within the walls of the meshwork lies the bone marrow. This delicate tissue contains vital populations of three types of immature cells: normoblasts, megakaryocytes, and white-cell precursors. Normoblasts proliferate and mature into oxygen-carrying red blood cells. Megakaryocytes produce platelets, to prevent hemorrhage at sites of minor trauma. The white-cell precursors mature to form infection-fighting lymphocytes and granulocytes. Most of the granulocytes are known as neutrophils and a smaller number form less important cells called eosinophils and basophils.

The mature forms of all these cells circulate in our bloodstream. By examining a sample of blood taken from a vein, we can calculate how many cells are present, and by examining them under a microscope we can see whether they appear normal. Acute leukemia strikes the marrow precursor cells. Although any of the precursors can be affected, the normoblasts and megakaryocytes are seldom involved, especially in children. The vast majority of childhood leukemias target the white-cell precursors, particular those producing lymphocytes. Primitive lymphocytes, known as lymphoblasts, divide and proliferate out of control. They take over the entire bone marrow and destroy other marrow residents. No bone is spared. The normal biochemical and physiological processes whereby a lymphoblast matures into an immunological useful lymphocyte are lost.

Instead of mature lymphocytes, a large number of immature lymphoblasts flood the bloodstream, raising the blood white-cell count up to ten or twenty times that seen in normal children. In a test tube, affected blood looks pale. This is what gives rise to the name leukemia (*leuk* = white, *emia* = blood). On rare occasions, the lymphoblasts remain trapped within the marrow and the patient has a very low white-cell count in the peripheral blood. This is termed aleukemic leukemia.

Apart from a rare form of T-cell leukemia, which affects patients in the Caribbean area and Japan, we do not know what causes childhood leukemia. As mentioned above, the Caribbean leukemia is caused by the HTLV1 (Human T Cell Leukemia Virus 1) retrovirus. While the hypothesis that many childhood leukemias might be virally induced is very attractive, we have insufficient data to incriminate viruses.

A few hereditary disorders predispose patients to leukemia. Children with Down's syndrome have about fifteen times the risk of normal children. A few other exceptionally rare conditions—such as ataxia-telangiectasia, congenital immunodeficiency, Fanconi's anemia, and Bloom's syndrome—also predispose to leukemia.

Rapid proliferation of primitive, immature white blood cells in the bone marrow characterizes acute leukemia. These spill into the peripheral blood, where they are readily detected. Leukemia is diagnosed by microscopic examination of blood and bone marrow. University hospitals and those hospitals affiliated with research protocols commonly use a comprehensive range of cell analyses to build a cytochemical and immunological profile of the leukemia cells.

Normal lymphocytes are classified as T-cells or B-cells according to various immunological properties. Lymphoblastic leukemias can also be subclassified as either T or B cell leukemias. However, a more useful classification is based on various microscopic and cytochemical parameters. The cytochemical features are identified microscopically after testing the leukemia cells with various chemicals. The commonest classification used is the French-America-British (FAB) classification. In the treatment of leukemia, and all other cancers, hematologists and oncologists try to adopt an internationally acceptable and uniform classification system. New treatments can then be tested worldwide and compared with older treatments, in the knowledge that like is being compared with like. Otherwise, different and confusing results may arise, because researchers will unknowingly share information on slightly different diseases, a bit like two friends discussing "Dave" without knowing they each have a different person in mind.

Because the cancerous white cells are immature, they do not function as normal white cells; they cannot protect against infection. Immunity is damaged or lost, and patients are susceptible to bacterial, viral, and fungal infections. Also, as the leukemia spreads through the marrow, it destroys the other normal cells. The result of platelet destruction is a tendency to spontaneously bleed into all tissues, but in particular into those tissues exposed to mild (often unrecognized) trauma, such as skin and mouth. Destruction of red blood cells leads to anemia. Anemic blood has a deficiency of the oxygen-carrying protein hemoglobin. The lack of oxygen, if severe enough, causes shortness of breath, a general lack of energy, and sometimes heart failure.

Intensive chemotherapy forms the mainstay of treatment. For many patients bone marrow or stem cell transplantation is also required.

Malignant lymphoma and Hodgkin's disease are discussed in chapter 6. One notable difference between adult and childhood lymphomas should be noted. In adults, there is a wide spectrum of non-Hodgkin's lymphoma types, ranging from low-grade indolent tumors to rapidly growing aggressive tumors. In children, almost all the non-Hodgkin's lymphomas are high-grade aggressive tumors.

As pointed out in chapter 6, there is an apparent paradox in the response of high-grade and low-grade lymphomas to treatment. Chemotherapy poisons many high-grade rapidly dividing lymphomas more easily than low-grade tumors. Most childhood lymphomas respond well to chemotherapy. Non-Hodgkin's lymphoma and leukemia in children are closely related pathologically, and treatment protocols are very similar.

Brain Tumors

Next in frequency, after leukemia and lymphoma, comes cancer of the central nervous system, i.e., the brain and spinal cord. We use neurons to see, hear, feel, move, and think. They are the nerve cells that control all important activities within the central nervous system. They live in the *gray matter* of the brain and spinal cord, surrounded and supported by another type of brain tissue called *white matter* and by a meshwork of supporting cells known as astrocytes. There are a variety of astrocyte subtypes, and tumors can arise from any of these cells or from primitive immature neurons. Neuropathologists classify brain tumors by their histopathological appearance, which reflects their cellular origin. Childhood brain tumors differ from those of adults in a number of ways. Most childhood astrocyte tumors (astrocytomas) are low-grade and amenable to surgical resection. They commonly involve that part of the brain at the back of the head called the cerebellum. Children with astrocytomas have a good chance of complete cure. In adults, astrocyte tumors involve various parts of the brain, are usually high-grade and aggressive, and are rarely curable. While tumors arising from neurons are rare in adults, they are relatively common in children. These are the medulloblastomas. They also arise in the cerebellum, and unlike the pediatric astrocytomas they are highly malignant.

While the histopathological classification gives us an indication of tumor aggressiveness, equally important is the size and location of the tumor. Size and location, along with the spread of tumor growth, determine what symptoms the child will have and whether the neurosurgeon will be able to remove it completely.

Brain tumors produce different symptoms in different patients. Any expanding growth within a rigid bony skull, irrespective of whether it is a tumor, an abscess, or a blood clot, will raise intracranial pressure. Raised intracranial pressure commonly causes severe headache and vomiting. The cerebellum, along with our eyes and inner ears, enables us to remain upright and walk in a straight line. Cerebellar tumors often cause loss of balance. Elsewhere in the brain tumors compress or damage signal pathways to the arms or legs, causing weakness or paralysis. Whey they damage pathways from the eye, they cause partial loss of vision. Some tumors destroy vision so slowly that neither the patients nor their parents are aware of altered eyesight. Special eye tests detect visual loss.

Not all brain tumors are malignant. Craniopharyngiomas, for example, arise just above the pituitary gland, from embryonic epithelial cells. Although craniopharyngiomas are benign, they sometimes invade the surrounding brain tissue, making them very difficult to remove completely. Tongues of incompletely removed tumor grow insidiously over the years and may need a second operation in adulthood. Meningiomas and neuromas are also benign and sit on the surface of the brain. The neurosurgeon can remove these with relative ease. Once a diagnosis of brain tumor is suspected, a CT or MRI scan quickly leads to the diagnosis. A small biopsy gives the definitive diagnosis, the classification, and the grade.

First-line treatment for childhood brain tumors is surgery. In some cases radiotherapy supplements it. In exceptional cases, it may be impossible to operate on a tumor because of its location. Chemotherapy has not played a major role in the treatment of childhood brain tumors up until recently. However, there is now evidence that some patients may benefit from chemotherapy. Special efforts are taken by radiotherapists and pediatric oncologists to minimize damage to the developing brain in young children. The great advances in the treatment of pediatric tumors have dramatically improved survival but have brought some serious long-term complications. For example, children under the age of eight are particularly at risk from whole-brain radiation. Studies carried out in the late 1980s and early 1990s showed that children who received such treatment often had a diminished IQ, subtle learning difficulties, and impaired socializing skills. Radiation to the areas surrounding the pituitary and a part of the brain called the hypothalamus often left children with endocrine deficiencies, due to lack of pituitary hormones. Awareness of these long-term complications will lead to therapeutic improvements in the future.

Wilms' Tumor

Abdominal cancers are next in frequency. One of these affects the kidneys and the other involves the adrenal gland, which sits on top of the kidney. Wilms' tumor (also less commonly known as nephroblastoma) is virtually never seen in adults. During embryonic and fetal development, the kidney evolves through various complicated stages until it becomes a mature kidney. Its principal function is to cleanse the bloodstream of various waste products that are toxic to other tissues. Using specialized epithelial cells, it produces urine and secretes the waste material. A network of connective tissue cells and tiny blood vessels enmeshes the epithelial cells. Wilms' tumor mimics primitive embryonic kidney tissue. It consists of a double population of epithelial cells and malignant connective tissue cells, called mesenchyme. Tumors of this kind, with two distinct neoplastic populations, are unusual and are said to have a biphasic growth pattern. Wilms' is usually sporadic (i.e., not familial or hereditary). However, a small percentage (1 percent) are familial. Almost 20 percent of familial Wilms' involve both kidneys. Bilateral involvement is unusual in the sporadic form and affects about 3 percent of patients.

The development of Wilms' appears to be caused by loss of one or more suppressor genes (see chapter 8). The best characterized is the WT1 (Wilms' Tumor Gene-1) on the short arm of chromosome 11. Genes on other chromosomes may also contribute to the onset and progression of Wilms'. Loss of genetic material located just alongside the Wilms' tumor gene causes two other rare syndromes, the Beckwith-Wiedemann and the Denys-Drash syndrome. Patients with either of these syndromes are at increased risk for Wilms' tumor. To discover at an early stage small, curable tumors, children with these rare syndromes are screened throughout their childhood by abdominal ultrasound examinations.

Frequently, Wilms' presents as a large abdominal swelling, usually before the age of four. The prognosis depends on tumor stage at the time of diagnosis. Like other staging systems, the various stages take into account whether the tumor is confined to the kidney or has spread outside the kidney, and how far it has spread. The microscopic appearance of the tumor is also of critical importance. Pediatric pathologists classify each tumor as having a favorable or unfavorable histology, depending on how aggressive it looks under the microscope. About 90 percent of patients have favorable histology (these are low-grade tumors). As well as stage and histology, patient survival rests on having access to a first-class pediatric oncology service. The best case is when a multidisciplinary team of experts, experienced in the diagnosis and treatment of this rare tumor, is available to handle predictable and unpredictable events that arise during the course of treatment.

Surgery, followed by chemotherapy, forms the mainstay of treatment. Some patients also have radiation treatment. The overall survival and cure rate for Wilms' is excellent, especially if it is diagnosed at a relatively early stage. For example, almost 45 percent of all patients are stage 1 at the time of diagnosis. Patients with stage 1 disease and favorable histology have a four-year survival rate of 97 percent. Most of these patients are completely cured.

A number of surveys in the past suggested that close relatives of children with cancer have an overall higher rate of cancer than the general population. A major study in 1995, in contrast, showed that parents of children with cancer are not at an increased risk.

Neuroblastoma

The second large cancer that grows intrabdominally in children is the neuroblastoma. It usually arises in the adrenal gland. We have two adrenal glands. Each sits on the upper pole of our kidneys, at the back of the abdominal cavity. The outer part of the adrenal, the cortex, secretes cortisol and a variety of related steroid hormones. It also secretes aldosterone, a hormone responsible for controlling fluid and salt balance and blood pressure. The cortex surrounds a specialized group of modified nerve cells in the adrenal medulla, and from these cells the neuroblastoma arises.

The normal adrenal medullary cells secrete epinephrine (adrenaline), norepinephrine, and a number of similar chemicals. Collectively, these are called catecholamines. Neuroblastoma tumor cells often retain their catechol-releasing powers and secrete these chemicals into the urine, where they can be detected. This provides the basis for a useful diagnostic test. Neuroblastomas are tumors of early childhood. Over 60 percent present before the age of five. They often present with a large abdominal mass, as in children with Wilms' tumor. However, they often metastasize early and may present with symptoms related to metastases, such as bone pain. About 70 percent of patients have metastases at the time of diagnosis. Sometimes patients present with some form of paraneoplastic syndrome, such as loss of balance. Paraneoplastic syndromes are due to a variety of metabolic abnormalities not related directly to either the bulk or physical mass of the primary tumor or the metastases. Paraneoplastic symptoms may affect patients with relatively small tumors and without metastases. Some of the symptoms are thought to be immunologically mediated. For instance, in patients with loss of balance, it is likely that antibodies against the tumor cells cross-react with some protein in the neurons of the cerebellum and somehow or other either destroy or interfere with neuronal function.

As in other cancers, prognosis depends to a large extent on stage at the time of diagnosis. However, neuroblastoma has one advantageous staging peculiarity, not shared by other cancers. If patients with disseminated disease have their metastases limited to skin, liver, or bone marrow and are under the age of one year, they have an excellent prognosis. These patients are classified as stage IV special (stage IVS). In addition to the usual features affecting prognosis, neuroblastomas have a number of molecular biology markers influencing prognosis. N-myc is a growth-promoting gene (a tumor oncogene); in some neuroblastomas this gene is amplified or reduplicated many times (up to 100 times normal). Tumors with highly amplified N-myc have a poorer prognosis than those without amplification. Similarly, an abnormal quantity of DNA (aneuploidy) in tumor cells often implies a bad prognosis.

Because most neuroblastomas secrete catechol amines, which appear in the urine, it is theoretically possible to screen young children for these tumors using a urine biochemical test. A number of studies in Japan, the United States, and the United Kingdom are investigating the overall value of such a screening program.

Treatment for neuroblastoma uses a combination of surgery and chemotherapy. Some patients also benefit from radiotherapy. Patients with localized, surgically resectable neuroblastoma have an excellent prognosis (even without chemotherapy). For patients with tumors at this stage, the cure rate is greater than 90 percent. For patients with disseminated disease, the long-term survival is 10 percent to 30 percent. The exception to this is the special category of stage IVS patients. This group has a 90 percent two-year survival, and most of these patients are cured.

Wonderful therapeutic advances also help cure many more patients with a variety of other less common pediatric cancers, such as retinoblastoma of the eye, Ewing's sarcoma, osteosarcoma of the bone, and soft tissue sarcomas of muscle and other connective tissues.

Nowhere has cancer success been more in evidence than in the field of pediatric oncology. Pediatric oncologists and hematologists have made spectacular advances during the past twenty years. Cancers that once were 100 percent fatal, such as acute leukemia and metastic neuroblastoma, are now curable in a high percentage of children. Overall, the prognosis for children with cancer is far better than for adults. Success in treating these cancers has followed decades of painstaking basic research in biochemistry, in molecular biology, and in pharmacology, followed by years of clinical trials. "Everything now known about curing a child with cancer," says the National Childhood Cancer Foundation, "has been learned from research." Adult oncologists look with envy at what their pediatric subspecialists have achieved and continue to achieve.

Bibliography

Bolande, R.P. Prenatal carcinogenesis. An appraisal. *Cancer* 74, 6 (1994):1674–79.

Ceballos, P.I., R. Ruiz Maldonado, and M.C. Mihm, Jr. Melanoma in children. *New England Journal of Medicine* 332, 10 (1995):656–62.

Coppes, M.J., D.A. Haber, and P.E. Grundy. Genetic events in the development of Wilms' tumor. *New England Journal of Medicine* 333, 9 (1994):586–90.

Cotran, R.S., V. Kumar, and S.L. Robbins. *Robbins pathologic basis of disease*. Philadelphia: Saunders, 1994.

Kase, L.M. Why community cancer clusters are often ignored. *Scientific American* 275 (1996):55–56.

La Vecchia, C., F. Levi, S. Franceschi, J.H. Olsen, J.D. Boice, Jr., N. Seersholm, A. Bautz, and J.F. Fraumeni, Jr. Screening for cancer, 1995: An update. *Annals of Oncology* 333, 24 (1995):1594–99.

Olsen, J.H., J.D. Boice, Jr., N. Seersholm, A. Bautz, and J.F. Fraumeni, Jr. Cancer in the parents of children with cancer. *New England Journal of Medicine* 333, 24 (1995):1594–99.

Pollack, I.F. Brain tumors in children. *New England Journal of Medicine* 331, 22 (1994):1500–07.

Richart, R.M., J.H. Olsen, J.D. Boice, Jr., N. Seersholm, A. Bautz, and J.F. Fraumeni, Jr. Screening. The next century. *Cancer* 333, 24 (1995):1594–9.

Internet Sources

Pediatric neuroblastoma: http://oncolink.upenn.edu/disease/neuroblast/
Pediatric Wilms' tumor: http://oncolink.upenn.edu/disease/ped-wilms/
Bone cancer: http://oncolink.upenn.edu/disease/bone1/
Pediatric Ewing's sarcoma: http://oncolink.upenn.edu/disease/ped-ewing/
Onco-link: Kids Corner: http://oncolink.upenn.edu/resources/kids/
Pediatric brain tumors: http://oncolink.upenn.edu/disease/ped-brain/
Pediatric leukemias: http://oncolink.upenn.edu/disease/leukemia/
General pediatric cancers: http://wwwicic.nci.nib.gov/pedpage/OtherSites.html
http://wwicic.nci,nib.gov/pedpage/OtherSites.html
http://www.pog.ufl.edu/publ/publ.html

CHAPTER 8

Genes and Cancer

The nucleus in each cell contains 46 chromosomes, arranged in 23 pairs. These are tightly wound, supercoiled, threadlike protein filaments; our genes reside on these threads. The 23 chromosome pairs (designated chromosomes 1 through 23) are not of equal length. Chromosome 1 is the longest and chromosome 21 is the shortest. If they were lined up end to end, the 46 chromosomes as they appear in usual microscopic preparations measure just 0.027 cm. However, if we uncoiled and straightened the chromosomes from just one nucleus they would measure six feet in length—amazing when you realize the diameter of one nucleus is approximately 10 microns (μm); stated another way, 100 cells add up to 1 millimeter (there are 1000 μm in 1mm). A 5,000 to 1 compaction ratio ensures that the 46 chromosomes can pack themselves into such a small space. Within the nucleus, genes are aligned along the chromosomes. Normally, in resting cells, the chromosomes lie tangled as threadlike chromatin. During mitosis, chromosomes separate, become discrete, and replicate before passing into daughter cells. The boxed area on the chromosome and the stars at the end of the tangled chromatin represent genes. These are composed of DNA.

Scientists first realized in 1950 that they could separate and study individual chromosomes. In the early days, microscopic chromosome preparations resembled a clump of dead worms—23 pairs, tangled, overlapped, and jumbled together. Biologists, in order to make any sense of them, photographed the mess, traced the outline of each chromosome, cut the outlines from the photographic print, and aligned the cutouts side by side. They called this photograph a karyotype. Each chromosome pair resembled a tiny doll with two outstretched arms and two legs. At that time, a standard nomenclature was adopted so that researchers around the world could communicate their new and exciting findings to each other. They classified chromosome groups as A, B, C, etc. on the basis of size and shape. Similar-appearing chromosomes were placed in the same group. Each chromosome pair has a constriction, like a tight waist. In some, the constriction (called a centromere) is exactly in the center. In others, it is located toward

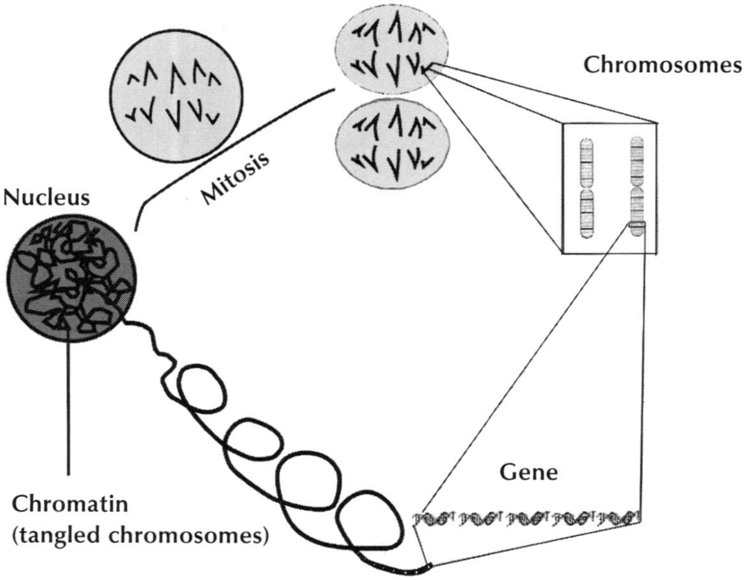

Figure 8.1. Nuclear chromatin.

one end. By convention, the shorter limbs (short arms) are called the p segments and the longer limbs (like legs but called long arms) are called the q segments.

Soon, doctors, especially pediatricians, realized that certain hereditary childhood disorders were associated with major chromosome abnormalities. They found that some children had too many and some had too few chromosomes in each cell. Sometimes large chunks of a chromosome were missing.

Advances in microscopy and staining techniques occurred rapidly. Certain dyes bound preferentially to different segments of each chromosome producing a highly characteristic banding pattern that allowed identification of each chromosome pair. Scientists devised a new, more accurate nomenclature, based on the banding technique. It was now possible to move away from just large A, B, C groups and to name each specific chromosome. Chromosome researchers now talk to each other in a language with a vocabulary containing chromosome numbers, p's and q's, band sizes, and specific band locations on the arms or legs. With the banding techniques, pediatricians found many more subtle abnormalities. In some diseases tiny fragments broke free from one chromosome and shifted to a different chromosome—these are translocations. Sometimes a small piece or even half of an entire chromosome might be flipped, inverted, and glued on backward to its original site.

Chromosome techniques and information progressed quickly, and soon a new medical laboratory technology emerged, cytogenetics. Specially trained technicians and doctors extracted useful genetic information from microscopic examination of abnormal chromosomes. Their early interests focused on hereditary disorders. Later, scientists applied the same techniques to cancer cells. While these advances moved at a rapid pace, a new science, molecular biology, was zooming along at breakneck speed. Molecular biologists had learned how to isolate and manipulate DNA, and their new techniques provided stunning insights into how genes control the normal cell. It is now evident that genetic damage is responsible for almost all the misguided properties of cancer cells.

James Dewey Watson and Francis Crick published the biochemical structure of DNA in 1953. It is a relatively simple structure, with its molecules arranged in a double helix. Chromosomes contain all genetic information embedded in a DNA code. The DNA helix is wound around a central protein core. DNA holds the biological secrets of life. Each gene consists of numerous groups of DNA (deoxyribonucleic acid) molecules. DNA, in turn, is composed in part from four chemicals called bases: (adenine, guanine, cytosine, and thymine, in figure 8.2).

How the bases (A, T, G, and C) are arranged in relation to each other determines most of our physical characteristics and how our body functions. The coded gene sequence is the blueprint for life. Bases are arranged in specific pairs; A always partners T, and C combines with G. The entire genetic makeup within the cell is the genome. Seven billion base pairs inhabit the 46 chromosomes—in every cell. Each base connects with an outer molecule of phosphate and a molecule of sugar called deoyribose. This combination of base, sugar, and phosphate is termed a nucleotide.

DNA, arranged in its double helix, resembles a spiral staircase or a twisted rope ladder. The outer side portion of the helix consists of the phosphate and deoxyribose. The central rungs are the bases. Each half of a rung consists of one base; this interlocks with its complementary base, making up the other half of the rung. As mentioned above, A locks with T and C locks with G, and each base pair makes one rung. Each group of three rungs codes for a single amino acid; amino acids are the building blocks from which proteins are made.

Distributed along the chromosomes are more than 100,000 functional genes. Between the functional units lie long segments of apparently inactive or "junk" DNA. Functional genes (exons) are ultimately responsible for directing protein synthesis and for our physical characteristics. The nonfunctional DNA segments are called introns, and these account for greater

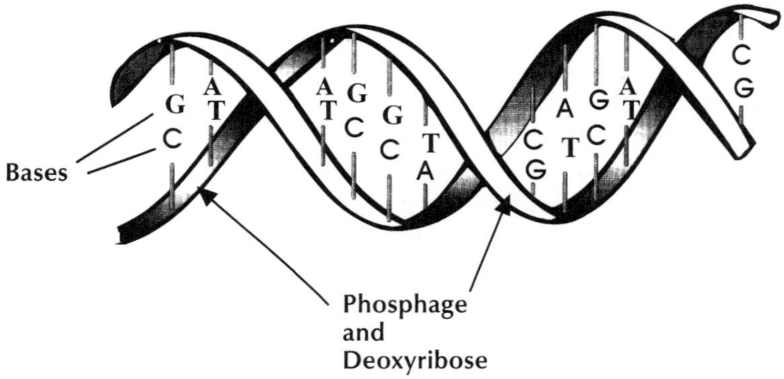

Figure 8.2. DNA

than 98 percent of all DNA. All humans have very similar DNA; each person's DNA differs from another's by only about 0.1 percent, or 3 million bases. These variations allow forensic scientists to use DNA for genetic fingerprinting. Remarkably, DNA makes up only about 0.3 percent of the total volume of the nucleus. Most of a cell's volume, like that of the entire body, consists of water. Like other cell components, the nucleus also contains a wide variety of peptides, proteins, and other life-supporting molecules.

DNA, the language of life, despite having only four letters (A, T, C, G), can write an infinite number of messages. At first, this statement might seem somewhat farfetched. After all, we need twenty-six letters to write in English. In fact, we need only two characters to write a complete language. Computers and digital equipment use binary code. They say everything with just two characters, 0 and 1. I typed this page of text on a computer keyboard using a word processor. The computer chip then converted each letter to binary code and delivered it to the screen, in English, and finally printed it on paper after being processed again through its two-character code.

To continue with this analogy to the English language, imagine that the genetic code is contained in an encyclopedia (the nucleus) consisting of 23 volumes (23 chromosome pairs). The *Encyclopædia Britannica* contains approximately 300 million letters. Each pair of chromosomes has about ten times as many letters. This means that we have approximately 3 billion letters in each cell, the equivalent of 200 Manhattan telephone books—200 books, each with a thousand pages. The human body contains more than 10 trillion (10^{13} cells) cells.

The English language has the most extensive vocabulary of any language. It is estimated that it contains more than 1 million words. Some other languages, such as Chinese, have a word-building capacity equal to that of English. The word-building capacity of the genetic code seems endless. Letters of the English language are strung together to form words. These in turn are woven into sentences, and finally the sentences are arranged in paragraphs. Spelling, grammar, and syntax govern how we write English. Likewise the language of the gene is arranged in amino acids (words), peptides (sentences), and proteins (paragraphs). Complicated syntax also controls their use. Unlike English words, the letters for each amino acid are all the same length (so too are those used by computer code); they consist of just three letters.

Our DNA alphabet encodes 26 amino acids. Each three-letter set is called a codon, and it encodes a single amino acid. The mathematics of using various three-letter codes from four possible letters means that there are sufficient letters for 64 amino acids. In fact, we have only 26 amino acids to construct every protein we possess; some of the code is redundant and a few identical amino acids are made by more than one codon. The cell then aligns these amino acids, joins them together like Lego pieces, and models them into three-dimensional proteins. Each instructing triplet (a codon) codes for one amino acid. Remarkably, the DNA code is the same in every living organism; bacteria and plants use the same DNA codes as humans.

How does this coding system work and what is its relevance to cancer? It functions like a feedback loop, similar to the flow of information from a computerized supermarket checkout to the stock inventory. As items move from the shelves or if there is an extra surge of customers, stocks become depleted. The bar-coded signals from checkouts order new items as required. When a cell requires new molecules of any type, or more protein, it sends a message to its nucleus. In response, the gene's DNA helix partially unzips down the middle, leaving its bases exposed. These bases rapidly form sticky templates as a sort of mold or model for the formation of another critical molecule, RNA (ribonucleic acid). A specific form of RNA, mRNA (messenger RNA), carries the message out into the cytoplasm and binds to ribosomes. These minifactories read the message and produce the required protein.

What happens if the computer develops a flaw or if the bar code sends a wrong signal? The supermarket might not get delivery or it might get a wrong item. A well-designed system will recognize an error and notify an operator, who will then correct the mistake. DNA also contains a diagnostic and self-correcting tool kit to identify and rectify many problems. Like a computer if its code is damaged, DNA will send the wrong message into the cytoplasm, possibly with disastrous consequences. Damaged DNA or a flaw in its code (a mutation) can bring a cell's metabolism to a sudden halt.

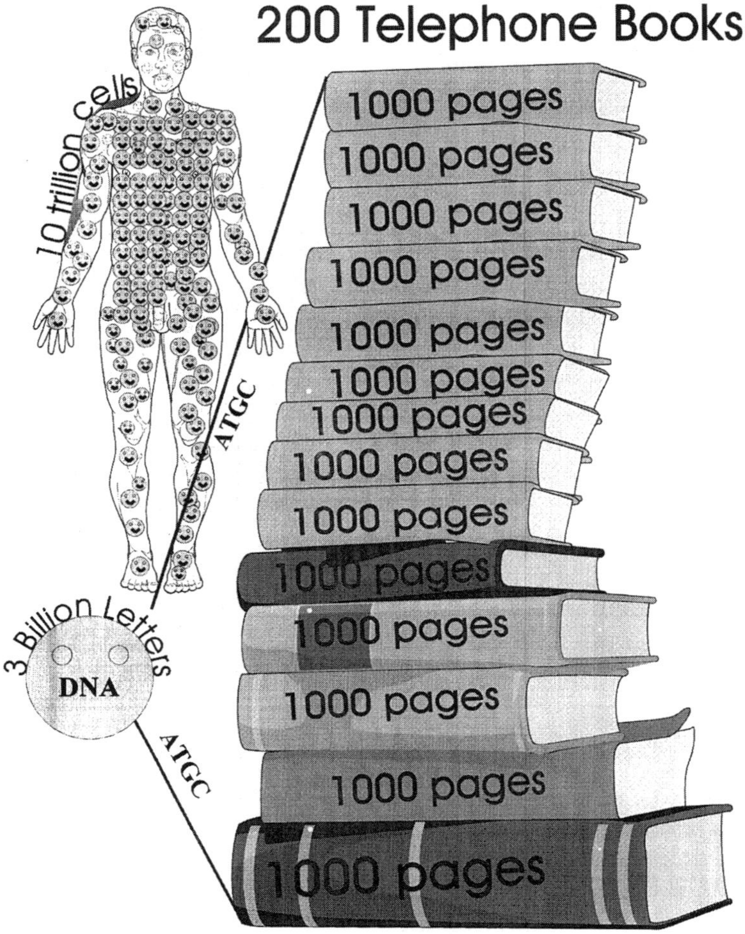

Figure 8.3. The DNA encyclopedia.

It might stop the cell from growing, make it grow more rapidly, let it accelerate out of control, or initiate any variety of other deviant behaviors. Loss of growth regulation is the essential abnormality in the cancer cell; this results from wrong DNA signals.

Apart from sending messages into the cytoplasm, DNA plays another crucial role. It controls cell replication. Each time a cell divides during mitosis, its DNA helix unzips completely, along the length of every chromosome. During cell division, an identical set of chromosomes with their genes is passed to the daughter cells. Before cell division takes place, the

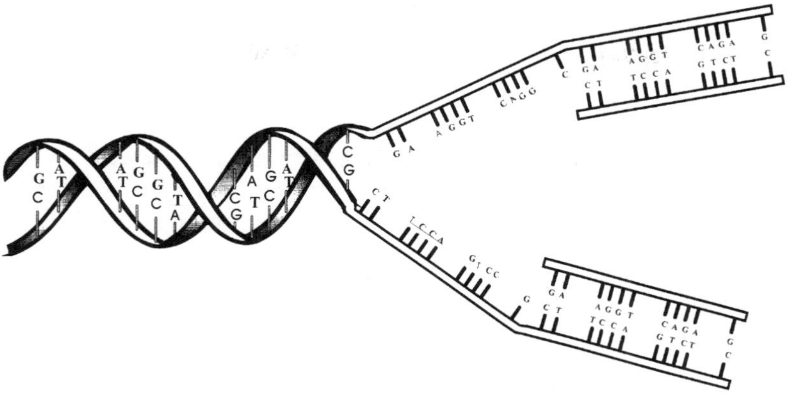

Figure 8.4. DNA replication.

DNA must replicate and produce an identical set of genes. All cells contain the same genes. However, different sets of genes are active in different cells and tissues. Each DNA strand, again acting as a template, binds a complementary set of ATGC bases to form a flawless replica of itself.

If the original cell contained a DNA mistake, the daughter cells contain the same mistake. The mistake is perpetuated in the offspring of all replicating cells. Some mistakes cause cancer.

Amino acids are the building blocks for all life's proteins, including enzymes, growth factors, and cell adhesion molecules. Genes vary in size (length) and are measured by the number of base pairs they contain. Each gene encodes a single protein or a major component of a protein. The genetic message passes from the nucleus through pores in the nuclear membrane into the cytoplasm. Here it binds to ribosomes, which are the factories responsible for gluing amino acids together to make protein. The messenger molecule is mRNA (messenger ribonucleic acid). The resultant proteins make their way to wherever they are needed. Sometimes they remain within the cell, and at other times they move into the bloodstream and travel to distant tissues.

The mechanisms whereby DNA self-replicates and encodes protein production are fine-tuned to an amazing degree. The slightest miscoding—such as occurs, for example, in sickle-cell anemia—can have disastrous consequences for the cell and its host. Our normal oxygen-carrying protein, hemoglobin, contains more than 500 amino acids. Hemoglobin is the main protein in our red blood cells. They are produced in abundance in the bone marrow every day and they have a life span of 120 days. Hemoglobin-coding genes faithfully replicate millions of times throughout our lives, and our ability to extract oxygen from the air we breathe depends on this process. In sickle-cell anemia, the patient's DNA has just one abnormally placed base in the hemoglobin-coding gene. This tiny mutation results in one abnormal amino acid substitution, in the sickle-cell hemoglobin. The resulting hemoglobin molecule (and the red blood cell) is distorted and misshapen and cannot release oxygen normally into tissues. As a result, the tissues suffer from chronic oxygen deprivation. In some patients this is fatal at an early age. Patients with a milder form of the disease survive into adulthood and transmit the same DNA deficiency to their offspring.

DNA abnormalities and genetic changes in epithelial cells also have disastrous consequences. Imagine a layer of breast epithelial cells sitting on a solid basement membrane. For years these divide and grow and die harmoniously, and in synchrony. They display a collective intelligence and respect each other's territory. Then something unknown silently starts to poison them, by interfering with the DNA helix. At first, the epithelium can ward off attacks. Even if the DNA is damaged, its built-in protective enzymes repair the helix, or if necessary, eliminate the damaged cell. However, after thousands of relentless and diversified sublethal attacks, minor DNA replication abnormalities appear in dividing cells. With each cell division the genetic abnormalities pass on to the daughter cells.

Eventually, a point of no return is reached; DNA repair mechanisms are exhausted. Once the replicating mechanism has been damaged, nearby DNA also becomes unstable. Like a snowball on a hill, alignment slippage along the helix gathers momentum and collects mutations at increasing frequency. After a few years the cells become dysplastic and are well on their way to becoming ductal carcinoma in situ (DCIS). In time, these changes affect genes controlling a variety of growth signals, and gradually the original cell and its daughters lose many of their normal growth-regulating mechanisms. This clone of abnormal cells now assumes some degree of independence and autonomy; it no longer grows and divides normally like its neighbors. As DNA defects continue to accumulate, the cell loses some functions and gains new, dangerous capabilities. Tumor cells eventually break through the basement membrane. Released from the confinement of the duct, they speed away, on their independent and relentless road to metastases.

A multitude of genetic and functional changes characterize cancer during its evolution. With the loss of self-regulating mechanisms, tumor cells assume some of the growth characteristics of cells in an early embryo. They are not differentiated and they secrete an array of growth-promoting factors and destructive enzymes. Furthermore, the cancer cells now acquire a sort of immortality and in experimental animals they become tumorigenic. If such cells are removed from the host and placed in an artificial cultural medium, they live and grow indefinitely. Even after the patient has died, these cells can continue to grow and divide in test tubes. Unlike cancer cells, normal cells in culture die after a limited number of cell divisions.

Scientists now think they understand why and how cancer cells achieve immortality. The ends of chromosomes are called telomeres, and they are critical in maintaining chromosomal integrity. Telomeres contain genes responsible for cell division and programmed cell death and function as molecular clocks. Daughter strands of DNA shorten with each DNA replication. Every time a cell divides, tiny telomere chunks are lopped off the end of the chromosome. Eventually, after a finite number of divisions, so much telomeric DNA is missing that the cells can no longer divide and multiply, and they die. This is part of the normal cell aging process.

Patients with progeria suffer from premature aging. In their teens they resemble, in every way, old age pensioners and are prone to all the ailments of old age. Progeria victims have profound shortening of their telomeres. Cancer cells, in their quest for immortality, protect their telomeres by producing an enzyme called telomerase, whose function is to stop the removal of telomeric DNA. This is one of the molecular tricks the cancer cell uses to prolong its survival.

About 90 percent of all cancers produce telomerase. In contrast, normal cells—apart from sperm and ova (eggs)—do not. Telomerase is not present in early cancers and so is not an important factor in their initiation. However, as cancer grows, telomerase appears and seems to be one of the factors responsible for tumor progression. If telomerase activity could be deactivated, cancer cells would die and tumor progression would halt. A number of research groups are struggling to find a telomerase inhibitor.

Mutations damage the DNA code and initiate the carcinogenic process. The sequence of words formed by the combination of ATGCs is very precise for every signal. Remove a T or add a G and you trick DNA into making the wrong amino acid. Put a wrong amino acid into a protein and it loses its function or possibly takes on a new function. For a harmless bacterium this could mean a new lease on life as a mutant killer. For a developing embryo it could mean eventual mental retardation, loss of an arm, or a crippling disease such as cystic fibrosis. For breast cells it might mean uncontrolled growth and cancer.

Scientists have cataloged a great many genetic defects in cancer cells. For convenience, we can categorize the relevant genes into three main groups, (1) oncogenes, (2) tumor suppressor genes, and (3) mismatch-repair genes. There are many types of mutations, almost all of which have a deleterious effect on the cell and its host. Oncogenes are growth-promoting genes that lie dormant, or function at a low rate, in normal differentiated cells but are overactive in the cancer cell. Their increased action can be likened to heavy pressure on an automobile accelerator. Tumor-suppressor genes are cellular brakes whose normal function is to regulate and slow growth. A combination of increased acceleration and loss of brakes is a recipe for disaster—uncontrolled growth. The cell speeds out of control. Mismatch-repair genes repair and realign minor DNA slippage. If these safety genes are damaged or inactivated, DNA mismatched during replication goes unchecked and accumulates relentlessly.

We have varying amounts of information concerning the structure, the location (on chromosomes), and the function of about 100 oncogenes. In normal cells they define orderly cell growth and maturation. It is only when they are overactive (overexpressed) that they cause problems. Sometimes, one particular oncogene may have a strong association with a particular cancer. The oncogene N-myc is frequently activated in childhood neuroblastomas, and those tumors with amplified N-myc activity are often more aggressive than those without amplification. However, N-myc may also be overexpressed in other malignancies, and so the abnormality is not specific for neuroblastoma. Commonly, a combination of oncogenes is overactive in cancers of all types.

Tumor suppressor genes have the opposite action to oncogenes; they slow down cell activity. Loss of suppressor genes increases cell growth from the unopposed action of proliferating signals. Each cell has a double dose of every gene. Individual genes are known as alleles; there are complementary alleles on the opposite limbs of each chromosome. Sometimes a particular function requires the activity of both alleles. At other times one allele takes charge and does all the work while its opposite number remains asleep and inactive. In the case of tumor suppressor genes, both are active and work in harmony. If one of them mutates, its partner assumes the responsibility of keeping the cell under control. If both mutate, this control is lost.

One tumor suppressor gene deserves special mention; it is called p53. Scientists have elevated p53 to almost hero status; in 1993 they voted it molecule of the year. Thousands of scientific papers document its structure and function and how it contributes to cancer growth. It lives on the short arm of chromosome 17. Here it may keep company with a number of notorious neighbors—rogue oncogenes and suppressor genes that commonly contribute to tumorigenesis. When it is healthy, this prima donna modulates many cell functions, including the rate of cell division and apoptosis. Mutated p53 loses these functions, turns delinquent, and becomes a villain.

The p53 gene interacts extensively with other controlling systems within the cell and modifies so many genetic processes that many scientists regard it as "the guardian of the genome." Although we do not understand all its functions, biologists have pinpointed a few of its key roles. It controls the beginning of the cell cycle and stabilizes cells in a resting state. When chemicals, radiation, or noxious proteins put a stress on normal cells, their natural tendency is to grow and proliferate, sometimes inappropriately; p53 stops inappropriate proliferation. Sometimes the chemical stimulation is too great and p53 cannot prevent cells from growing and dividing. Under such circumstances it turns ruthless—it kills them and prevents abnormal growth. In its managerial and supervisory rules, it instructs some of its helpers to activate suicide genes and these induce apoptosis. It also contributes to the machinery responsible for DNA repair. Mutated p53 loses these protective properties, and cells proliferate out of control.

More than 50 percent of all cancers show p53 mutations; these include the common cancers—breast, lung, prostate, and colon. The p53 mutations are the commonest genetic changes in cancer. Some cancer-prone families have inherited p53 mutations. Best studied is the Li-Fraumeni syndrome. Patients with this syndrome get early-onset breast cancer, childhood sarcomas, and other cancers. Individuals with inherited p53 mutations have a 50 percent chance of getting cancer before the age of 30 and this risk increases to nearly 90 percent by the age of 65. Fortunately, the Li-Fraumeni syndrome is rare. Loss of p53 protective function leaves tissue susceptible to the carcinogenic effects of chemotherapy and radiotherapy, which leaves patients at risk for treatment-induced second cancers. The p53 gene encodes a critical protein (p53 protein), and it is this protein that directs much of the cell's growth. Despite intense investigation, neither the gene nor its protein have yielded all their secrets.

Molecular evolution favors survival of the fittest. For those tumor cells unable to make or find new blood vessels (see chapter 5—angiogenesis), mutations in the p53 oncogene confer the advantage of requiring little or no oxygen. By clonal growth tumor cells with far lower requirements for oxygen and nutrition can proliferate happily.

As mentioned earlier, another area of intense research is the control of programmed cell death—apoptosis. Normal growth requires a balance between cell growth, differentiation, survival, and death. Two families of proteins play key roles as positive regulators in this balance; these are the cyclins and cyclin-dependent kinases (CDK). The negative regulators are tumor suppressor proteins and the newly discovered CDK inhibitors (CDKI). The positive regulators allow the cell to pass through the various checkpoints in the cycle, whereas the negative regulators keep the positive regulators from proceeding too quickly. The real secret, still waiting to be discovered, is how exactly all these regulators interact intelligently with each other.

A large proportion of basic cancer research is focused on this topic of growth regulation. One of the CDKIs is a protein named p21. The gene controlling p21 is a master switch gene, it helps regulate the cell's decision to divide or differentiate. The p21 protein sits at the center of a hub of activity, modifying DNA synthesis, cell division, differentiation, and apoptosis. Recent research indicates that low p21 production causes cell-cycle progression, whereas increased production stops the cell cycle and switches the cell to a differentiation mode.

Suicide genes, using a number of biological mechanisms, assist the process of normal cell regulation. They trigger apoptosis in some tumors but not in others. Tumors showing a good apoptotic response are frequently chemosensitive and respond well to chemotherapy, and they have an excellent prognosis. The p53 gene appears to play an important role here also, by modulating the apoptotic response. Tumors with mutated p53, unable to respond with apoptosis, resist chemotherapy and radiotherapy.

DNA repair genes, like p53, help to maintain the integrity of the genome. These recently recognized genes (also called DNA mismatch-repair genes), patrol the DNA double helix. Minor errors appear continuously along the DNA molecule. Unchecked, these would translate into injurious signals, leading to abnormal growth and cell division. One eminent researcher calculated that up to 1 billion tiny DNA errors take place every time a cell divides. The mismatch repair system proofreads the DNA code. When it finds an error, it changes the code to the correct one or snips a strand of damaged DNA and replaces it with a small length of correct DNA. Mutations in the mismatch-repair genes contribute to some forms of cancer. For example, hereditary mutations in DNA repair genes are responsible for about 10 percent of colon cancers.

Cancer specialists and scientists are now certain that gene mutations, deletions, or rearrangements lie at the heart of cancer initiation and progression. An alternative theory, not widely held, is that mutations are a secondary event. This latter hypothesis suggests that some, as yet unknown, process initiates tumorigenesis and as a result of abnormal cell growth the mutations observed by molecular biologists are a secondary effect. However, the overwhelming evidence indicates that damaged genes are responsible for tumor initiation and progression.

Carcinogens may sometimes inflict injury far more impressive than subtle gene mutations. Sometimes an entire chromosome or one of its limbs, with thousands of genes, is deleted from the nucleus. At other times a large fragment breaks from one chromosome and grafts itself onto another chromosome (a translocation). Such chromosomal abnormalities are common in many cancers. Sometimes a specific translocation is characteristic of one type of cancer.

Chronic myeloid leukemia (CML) is one of the commoner types of adult leukemia. In CML, the white blood cells show a specific translocation from chromosome 9 to chromosome 22. The abnormal chromosome 22 is called the Philadelphia chromosome and has diagnostic and prognostic significance. This translocation is so large that cytogeneticists can see it microscopically, and hematologists have known of its existence since 1968, before the molecular biology revolution. With the advent of sophisticated molecular biology techniques, it became evident that the split in chromosome 9 always occurs at the same site, where the oncogene *abl* and *bcr* is in some way responsible for the initiation of CML. Experimental evidence supports this hypothesis, as CML can be induced in rats by artificially translocating *abl* to *bcr.*

The greatest biology project of all time, The Human Genome Project, equivalent to or greater than any space project, started in 1990 and will finish in the year 2005; already the project is ahead of schedule. The National Institutes of Health and the U.S. Department of Energy distribute most of the funding. When this $3 billion venture ends, we will have a map of every human gene, its chromosomal address, and its genetic code. We will know where the genes contributing to more than 4,000 diseases are located and what they look like.

The purpose of this mammoth project is to map every gene and to sequence the entire human genome. There are about 5,000 genes located on each chromosome; each gene has an average of about 30,000 base pairs. The estimated 100,000 genes make up only 5 percent of our total DNA, and these are hidden in a jungle of similar genetic material which until recently was considered to be silent and was often referred to as "junk DNA." We now know that these hidden sequences may have important roles in protecting the genes. The genome researchers will catalog and sequence the 3 billion bases that make up the genome. Laboratories throughout the world contribute to this extravaganza, and in these laboratories, geneticists collaborate with biologists, biochemists, computer programmers, and robotics experts. To bring this project to fruition, the organizational skills of team leaders will be almost as important as their research ingenuity.

Much of the information from the genome project will be relevant to cancer researchers. Cancer specialists believe that the secrets of abnormal cell behavior lie in our understanding of the genetic mechanisms controlling normal cells. When we understand these mechanisms, we will have a better insight into the workings of the cancer cell. The mysteries of the cell cycle, apoptosis, the cell's adaptive response to an adverse environment, and cell-to-cell signaling will be revealed. In due course, this knowledge will open doors for many new treatments, including gene therapy.

Bibliography

Aas, T., A.L. Borresen, S. Geisler, B. Smith Sorensen, H. Johnsen, J.E. Varhaug, L.A. Akslen, and P.E. Lonning. Specific p53 mutations are associated with de novo resistance to doxorubicin in breast cancer patients. *Nature Medicine*, 2, 7 (1996):811–14.

Albelda, S.M. Role of integrins and other cell adhesion molecules in tumor progression and metastasis. *Laboratory Investigations* 68, 1 (1993):4–17.

Axelrod, N. Of telomeres and tumors. *Nature Medicine* 2, 2 (1996):158–59.

Batsakis, J.G., and A.K. El-Naggar. p53: Fifteen years after discovery. *Advances in Anatomic Pathology* 2 (1995):71–88.

Berns, A. Is p53 the only real tumor suppressor gene? *Current Biology* 4 (1994):137–39.

Bishop, G.E., and M. Waldholz. *Genome.* New York: Touchstone, 1990.

Bishop, J.M., and R.A. Weinberg. *Scientific American molecular oncology*. New York: Scientific American Medicine, 1996.

Boguski, M.S., J.H. Olsen, J.D. Boice, Jr., N. Seersholm, A. Bautz, and J.F. Fraumeni, Jr. Hunting for genes in computer data bases. *New England Journal of Medicine* 333, 24 (1995):1594–99.

Brash, D.E. Cellular proofreading. *Nature Medicine* 2, 5 (1996):525–26.

Cotran, R.S., V. Kumar, and S.L. Robbins. *Robbins pathologic basis of disease.* Philadelphia: Saunders, 1994.

Folkman, J. Seminars in Medicine of the Beth Israel Hospital, Boston, Clinical applications of research on angiogenesis. *New England Journal of Medicine* 333, 26 (1995):1757–63.

Gribbin, J. *In search of the double helix.* London: Corgi Books, 1991.

Harris, C.C., and M. Hollstein. Clinical implications of the p53 tumor-suppressor gene. *New England Journal of Medicine* 329, 18 (1993):1318–27.

Judson, H.F. *The eighth day of creation. Makers of the revolution in biology*. London: Penguin Books, 1995.

Keoles, D.J., and L. Hood. *The code of codes: scientific and social issues in the human genome project.* Cambridge, Mass., II Harvard University Press, 1991.

Kinzler, K.W., and B. Vogelstein. Cancer therapy meets p53. *New England Journal of Medicine* 331, 1 (1994):49–50.

Lindahl, T. DNA repair. DNA surveillance defect in cancer cells. *Current Biology* 4, 3 (1994):249–51.

Marx, J. DNA repair comes into its own. *Science* 266, 5186 (1994):728–30.

_____. New link found between p53 and DNA repair. *Science* 266, 5189 (1994):1321–22.

Milner, J. DNA damage, p53 and anticancer therapies. *Nature Medicine* 1 (1995):879–80.

Pennisi, E. New gene forges link between fragile site and many cancers. *Science* 272 (1996):649.

Pietenpol, J.A., and B. Vogelstein. Tumor suppressor genes. No room at the p53 inn. *Nature* 365, 6441 (1993):17–18.

Rabbitts, T.H. Chromosomal translocations in human cancer. *Nature* 372, 6502 (1994):143–49.

Rubin, E., and J.L. Farber. *Pathology*. Philadelphia: J.B. Lippincott, 1994.

Ruoslahti, E. How cancer spreads. *Scientific American* 275 (1996):42–47.

Shapiro, R. *The human blueprint.* London: Cassell Books, 1991.

Steller, H. Mechanisms and genes of cellular suicide. *Science* 267, 5203 (1995):1445–49.
Weinberg, R.A. The cell cycle clock and cancer. *Scientific American* 275 (1996): 36–37.
Wills, C. *Exons, introns, and talking genes.* New York: Basic Books, 1991.
Wright, P.A., and D. Wynford-Thomas. Mutations in familial cancer. 172 (1994): 167–70.
Wyllie, A.H. Apoptosis. Death gets a brake. *Nature* 369, 6478 (1994):272–73.
Young, S. Life and death in the condemned cell. *New Scientist* 25 (Jan. 1992):34–37.

CHAPTER 9

What Causes Cancer?

"How is it that we put a man on the moon more than thirty years ago and we still have not found a cure for cancer?" is a question patients frequently ask doctors. We will never conquer cancer until we discover what is causing it. Although we may have wonderful diagnostic tests and new treatments, we will continue to play a catchup game until we can identify and eliminate the cause. Is it feasible or realistic to think we can conquer cancer? Not in the immediately foreseeable future. Why? Cancer is not a single disease. It is a group of more than a hundred similar ailments that we lump together under one name, and we do not know what causes most of them. Because cancer is not a single disease, it is inconceivable that all cancers could have the same cause.

Although we have little insight into the causes of many of the common cancers, we are not totally ignorant. Let's begin by asking "how do we know what causes any cancer?"

First, someone assumes guilt by association and makes a theoretical link between some type of cancer and a possible cause. Initially, this link is based on a clinical observation. In 1775, a London surgeon, Percivall Pott, observed a high incidence of scrotal cancer in chimney sweeps. He hypothesized that prolonged contact with ingrained soot in their trousers might be causing these cancers. He was right. He did not understand the chemical composition of the various carcinogenic tars in soot. Nevertheless, he was able to eliminate this form of skin cancer by getting the chimney sweeps to improve their hygiene by frequent washing and by protecting the scrotal skin from prolonged soot exposure. Something in the soot brought on the cancer. This was the first link between a specific occupational cancer and chemical carcinogenesis. Before this discovery, doctors thought chronic irritation caused scrotal cancer.

Hardly a day passes but the newspapers, radio, or television tell us that researchers have found a link between some chemical, hormone, activity, or whatever, and cancer. We have almost reached an anxiety-of-the-week syndrome. Often, reports are conflicting. A major study in the *New Eng-*

land Journal of Medicine (a highly prestigious and reliable medical journal) reported in August 1990 that there was a strong link between coffee intake and cancer of the pancreas. In 1993 another major study showed that there was no link. Little wonder that the public is confused. How do these reports come about? Why does one group of investigators get different results from another? How can we know who to believe?

Let's look at how these reports arise. Almost invariably, epidemiologists carry out these studies. Epidemiologists are medical doctors or scientists trained in biostatistics who analyze information recorded in patients' charts, company records, or responses to questionnaires. They do not carry out laboratory experiments to show that such-and-such a substance causes cancer. Unlike laboratory scientists, epidemiologists have relatively few sophisticated methods for assessing quality assurance. They have no laboratory procedures for calibrating equipment or for measuring the direct effects of toxic substances on animals, tissues, or cells. Epidemiology is an observational science, concerned with measuring the association between risk factors and disease. They examine circumstantial evidence, looking for links between what we eat, drink, and breathe in our environment and disease. They also quantify this risk. The questions they ask are important and relevant. In recent times epidemiologists have been the heroes in identifying cigarettes, asbestos, and polyvinyl chloride as cancer-causing culprits.

Epidemiological tools include randomized trials, case control studies, and cohort studies. The randomized trial is a powerful study method and highly reliable. Such trials are now standard for evaluating new or controversial medical and surgical treatments. However, they are not practical for assessing epidemiological risk-factor studies. Randomized trials are prospective studies with each study variable planned in detail. They usually involve multiple centers, often in many countries, on different continents. Hundreds of thousands of individuals are frequently required for each study. It may take a decade or even longer to generate data for analysis.

With case control studies two groups are compared. One group of patients, with a specific disease, is questioned in detail about daily activities, and their responses are compared to those of a control group without the disease. A cohort study is more reliable than the case control study but is also more costly. A large population is required, often as many as 100,000. These subjects have no disease at the time the study begins. They fill in a detailed questionnaire and are followed up for decades to see who gets sick and who doesn't and what factors might be correlated with disease. Much of the information we have about the relationship between heart disease and lifestyle comes from such long-term cohort studies. Apart from the logistic problems of needing a huge number of study subjects and long time intervals, there are inherent problems with the design of and responses to questionnaires. Responses are often unreliable, especially when results depend on something such as human memory. Epidemiologists are conscious of the vagaries and limitations of biases and confounding factors, and they try to eliminate as many of them as possible. A classical confounding variable is the association between cigarette smoking and alcohol intake. It would be foolish to think that one could study alcohol ingestion without allowing for the possibility that smoking and alcohol go hand in glove and one could study neither in isolation. Such confounding links are not always so easy to spot.

Therefore, when you hear that some famous university researchers have just discovered a link between some activity and cancer, how do you know whether it is important? Experts recommend some useful guidelines. Cohort studies are more reliable than case control studies. Risk factors for people exposed are expressed as a ratio to the normal population, and the normal ratio is one. Risk ratios less than 3 are not, in general, very reliable. Such ratios may be due to the methodology used and not a true result. Credible risk ratios should be greater than 4. Furthermore, the conclusion should make some biological sense. Before the results are accepted, subsequent studies should confirm the first results. Preferably the subsequent studies would use different questions or methodology to arrive at the same conclusions. Otherwise the same biases might creep into both studies.

Sometimes it is possible to get supporting evidence from laboratory studies. In general, epidemiological studies can easily tell big differences from little differences. However, it is difficult to tell the difference between what is normal and a small result. Small differences may nevertheless be very important when they apply to millions of people.

Scientists can cause unnecessary panic. For example, they might show that some chemical causes cancer in rats and then this cause and effect is unjustifiably applied to humans. However, humans are not rats, and a chemical in one species may have different consequences in another. Furthermore, they may expose the rats to huge doses of the carcinogen—doses that humans are never likely to experience. Such was the case with the sweetener saccharin. In the early 1970s, scientists found that enormous quantities of saccharin could cause bladder cancer in rats. Despite numerous studies showing that the sweetener does not cause human cancer, the association still lingers in the public's mind. Advertisers of other sweeteners, who state that their product "does not contain saccharin," sometimes subtly reinforce and perpetuate this idea.

Most doctors feel that the news media report cancer risks inaccurately, often out of context and sometimes irresponsibly. Journalists often blow findings out of proportion and do not explain to the public the limitations of the studies. It could also be argued that researchers, universities, and research institutes are frequently just as guilty. There is often a great temptation to try to give one's research more importance than it deserves, and researchers may give biased or slanted information to journalists at press releases. The reader should take much of what he or she reads in the lay press about new cancer risks with a good grain of salt.

To organize our ideas, we can begin by stratifying the causes of cancer into two main risk groups: (1) those cancers caused primarily by environmental conditions, and (2) those cancers with a strong hereditary predisposition.

Environmental Factors

Since most adult cancers have no known hereditary predisposition, epidemiologists postulate that carcinogens in the environment cause most cancers. We can group the culprits in our environment into a few major groups, such as chemicals, radiation, and viruses. For many years the causal relationship between certain cancers and noxious chemicals in the workplace has been clear. Tighter public health regulations have eliminated most of these chemicals. Dye workers got cancer of the bladder from naphthylamine. Workers exposed to asbestos fibers got malignant mesotheliomas of the pleura (the outer lining of the lung). Those exposed to polyvinylchloride got angiosarcomas of the liver. Natives of central Africa got liver cancer from aflatoxins produced by a fungus growing on their food. Where the incidence of gastric cancer is high it is likely that chemicals associated with food processing are the cause.

Table 9.1 Cancers Caused by Chemicals

Chemical	Source	Cancer Type
Polycyclic hydrocarbons	Cigarette smoke larynx, esophagus, bladder, possibly others	Lung, mouth, throat,
Vinyl chloride	Plastics industry	Liver cancer
Aflatoxin	Food contaminant	Liver cancer in Africa
Napthylamine	Dye industry	Bladder cancer
Nitrosamines	Smoked food	Cancer of the stomach
Asbestos*	Shipbuilding and insulation industries	Mesothelioma of the lung
Chemotherapy drugs	Anticancer drugs	Leukemia

** Strictly speaking, asbestos is not a chemical. It consists of various fibers, some of which are more carcinogenic than others.*

Some experts believe that dietary factors are responsible for up to 30 percent of all cancers in the western world. These include animal fats, salt and alcohol. Lack of vegetables and fruit in our diet may also be a contributing factor. Despite their bad publicity in the past, we know that neither coffee nor artificial sweeteners cause cancer.

Probably the best-known carcinogens are the polycyclic aromatic hydrocarbons found in cigarette smoke. Experimentally, these chemicals produce cancers in a wide variety of tissues. Their main link is with lung cancer. Everyone, with the possible exception of some tobacco companies, accepts that smoking causes lung cancer. Epidemiologists argue that cigarette smoking may contribute to 30 percent of all cancer deaths (and 21 percent of all cardiovascular deaths). Although we know the cause of the greatest cancer killer of all, i.e., lung cancer, smokers continue to puff away apparently oblivious of the nightmare ahead of them. Other well-known chemical carcinogens are vinyl chloride, aflatoxin, aromatic amines and azodyes, nitrosamines, some metals, and surprisingly, some anticancer chemotherapeutic drugs.

Chemical carcinogenesis has been studied extensively in animal models and cell culture systems. It is a multistep process often requiring a number of chemicals acting in combination or in sequence. The terms *initiation* and *promotion* are commonly used. The initiator begins the process, but on its own will not lead to cancer. The promoter will not cause cancer until tissue has been primed by the initiator.

Factors that may influence the susceptibility to chemical carcinogens include the sex and hormonal status of an individual. Early and frequent pregnancies appear to have a protective effect against cancer of the breast, endometrium (the lining of the uterus), and ovary. Early menarche (first onset of periods) and late menopause increase the risk for cancer in these organs. Perhaps it is the prolonged lifetime of exposure to female hormones that increases the risk. Breast cancer is rare in males. Epidemiologists do not understand why pregnancy is protective. One hypothesis is that it somehow enhances tissue differentiation, especially in the breast, and that this differentiation has a protective effect.

We live in a polluted world. Intuitively, most reasonable people would expect that the filth in the air that we citydwellers breathe must be a major cause of cancer. Surprisingly, there is little evidence that this is so. The experts reckon that pollution contributes up to only 2 percent of fatal cancers, mostly lung and bladder. Ecologists tell us that urban smokers are more likely to get lung cancer than their rural cousins. Yet urban nonsmokers are not at increased risk. It appears that long-term exposure to high levels of air pollution increases the risk of lung cancer in smokers by up to 50 percent. This is a relatively small risk when taken in the context of heavy smoking itself; compared to nonsmokers, heavy smokers have a 2,000 percent risk. It is obvious that some people are relatively resistant to the carcinogenic action of many chemicals. Possibly these people have the necessary genetic machinery to inactivate or detoxify those injurious chemicals.

Some tissues are in constant contact with the external environment, and it is easy to understand how environmental carcinogens affect them. Ultraviolet (UV) radiation bombards our skin. The more UV radiation we receive, the more likely we are to get skin cancer. Likewise, it is not too difficult to imagine that carcinogens in inhaled air deliver maximum damage to the lining of lung and that ingested carcinogens damage the lining of the intestine. Cancers of the lung and intestine arise mostly from the lining epithelium of these tissues. However, it is more difficult to visualize how environmental carcinogens cause breast or prostate cancer, and we have no definite evidence that they do. Nevertheless, it is well known that some chemicals are not carcinogenic until they have been modified. Perhaps some environmental toxins attack the breast and prostate after modification. Modification may take place in the liver by certain chemical actions.

Sometimes chemicals have a direct carcinogenic effect; others have an indirect effect. One chemical with a direct effect is the chemotherapeutic drug Busulphan. Chemotherapeutic drugs are lifesavers for cancer patients. Paradoxically, some drugs like Busulphan may induce a new cancer many years after the original cancer has been cured. Radiation therapy has a similar oncogenic effect on some patients. Some chemicals are not directly carcinogenic. The body breaks them down into toxic metabolites, and it is the metabolites that are carcinogenic. Such is the situation with aniline dyes, which break down into a metabolite which is responsible for bladder cancer. Before aniline was recognized as a carcinogen, aniline dye workers had a high incidence of bladder cancer. Many researchers feel it is only a matter of time before we will discover that other unrecognized chemicals in our food and in our environment are responsible for many common cancers.

In certain geographical regions some cancers are particularly common, and the question that frequently arises is whether the people native to that region have a genetic predisposition to develop this type of cancer or whether it is something in their environment. The mortality rate for stomach cancer in Japan is approximately seven times that in the United States. However, when the Japanese immigrate to the United States their offspring have a mortality rate from gastric cancer similar to Caucasian Americans. Such epidemiologic information provides strong evidence that the cause of their cancer is in the environment. Other epidemiological migrant studies provide similar evidence about colon cancer.

Physical agents such as radiation and asbestos cause cancer. The cancer-producing effects of radiation are well documented. Hiroshima and Nagasaki survivors had a high incidence of leukemia. Ionizing radiation is carcinogenic, whether in the form of electromagnetic radiation such as X rays or gamma rays, or particulate radiation in the form of alpha or beta particles, protons or neutrons. Early pioneers in the development of X rays, including Marie Curie, got radiation-induced cancers. Early diagnostic radiologists, before they learned to protect themselves from radiation, often got leukemia, as did ankylosing spondylitis patients who had their spinal inflammation treated by radiation. Ankylosing spondylitis is an unusual form of spinal arthritis that often responded dramatically to radiotherapy. In the early 1950s infants with large thymuses had these organs shrunken with radiation therapy. The thyroid gland was usually included in the radiation field. Subsequently, many patients developed thyroid cancer. Already we have a surge of thyroid cancers from the Chernobyl disaster in 1986. The number of predicted future cancer deaths from this nuclear disaster ranges from 6,500 to 45,000.

Table 9.2 Cancers Caused by Radiation

Type of Radiation	Source	Cancer Type
Ultraviolet radiation	Sun	Skin cancers: squamous and basal cell, melanoma
Electromagnetic radiation	Radiotherapy machines	Sarcomas at radiated site. Thyroid cancer
Radioisotopes, e.g., Thorotrast	Nuclear fallout Used to improve X-ray visualization in the past	Thyroid cancer, leukemia, liver and bone cancer

In the 1950s radiologists examined patients with the aid of a radioactive drug called Thorotrast. This substance remained sequestered in the liver for the rest of the patient's life. Many patients got liver cancer years later. Patients treated for various cancers with high dose radiotherapy ran the risk of developing a new cancer about ten years later, at the site of the previous radiation. Other well documented examples of radiation-induced cancers include lung cancer in uranium miners who inhaled radioactive dusts and workers who painted radium-containing material onto watches to create luminous dials. This latter group had the habit of licking their paint brushes to produce a fine point; they absorbed the radioactive radium.

An unresolved question about low-level radiation in our environment is how much it contributes to cancer. The "no threshold hypothesis" states that radiation doses have no safe cutoff point. Recently it has become evident that granite in some geographical regions gives off high levels of radon gas. This results from uranium and radium decay in the ground. The products of radon bind to dust in homes located in these regions. This is then inhaled and deposited in the lungs. Approximately 4 percent to 5 percent of United States homes have radon levels at least 5 times the average background level. Despite the natural and very understandable fears of residents in these areas, the significance of radon exposure in the home is still hotly debated and unresolved. Recently, the "no threshold hypothesis" has been challenged. The idea that radiation is carcinogenic, no matter how small the dose, is based on mutation studies on fruit flies, carried out in 1927. More recent studies suggest that the risk may not be linearly related to dose. In fact, there may be threshold levels below which radiation is not carcinogenic.

Ultraviolet radiation is another form of radiation and is produced by the sun. Ultraviolet rays are classified according to their wavelength. It is now clear that ultraviolet B is responsible for about 90 percent of the common skin cancers, basal cell and squamous cell carcinomas. In some patients it also plays a major role in the causation of malignant melanomas. Fair-skinned people, especially the freckled Celtic races, are particularly at risk for developing all forms of skin cancer. If they live in sunny climates, such as Australia, they are particularly susceptible. In contrast, darkly pigmented skin provides good protection from sun-induced skin cancer.

Considerable controversy surrounds the malignant properties of non-ionizing electromagnetic fields, such as those near high-voltage electric lines. Although the experts have not dismissed the possibility, at present there is no convincing evidence that electromagnetic fields cause cancer. Likewise, despite disturbing reports in our news media from time to time, we have little concrete evidence that microwaves or ultrasound waves cause cancer.

Asbestos is another well-documented cancer-causing substance. Once inhaled, asbestos remains in our lungs forever. About 2 percent to 3 percent of exposed workers get an unusual form of cancer called malignant mesothelioma. This malignancy destroys the outer lining of the lung (pleura). Continued long-term exposure is not necessary. Mesothelioma typically develops after a long latent period (the interval between exposure and the onset of cancer), often up to twenty years, sometimes after much longer intervals. Spouses and other people living in the same house as asbestos workers have also developed mesothelioma, presumably from inhaled asbestos fibers from the workers' clothes.

Viruses are implicated in a small number of cancers. In central Africa, the Epstein-Barr virus is strongly associated with Burkitt's lymphoma and probably plays an important part in its causation. The same virus is responsible for glandular fever, also known as infectious mononucleosis or the kissing disease. Burkitt's lymphoma is a high-grade, rapidly proliferating cancer of lymphocytes (lymph node cells and white blood cells responsible for our immune protection). Most of the population of the western world show, in blood tests, evidence of previous infection—even if they had no clinical evidence of infectious mononucleosis in the past. Subclinical infections are quite common with a wide variety of viruses. These patients show no ill effects for the rest of their lives. The same virus frequently colonizes a number of other cancers, in particular cancer of the throat, in China. However, its precise relationship to cancer is still unknown.

Table 9.3 Cancers Caused by Viruses*

Type of Virus	Cancer Type
Papilloma virus (HPV)	Cancer of the cervix
Epstein-Barr virus (EBV)	Burkitt's lymphoma (Africa), nasopharyngeal carcinoma (China), possibly other lymphomas
Hepatitis B virus (HBV)	Liver cancer (Asia and Africa)
HTLV1	Leukemia, lymphoma (Caribbean, Japan)

**There is much evidence implicating these viruses as carcinogenic agents. We await final proof.*

The HTLV1 virus is closely linked to one unusual type of leukemia, with a high incidence in Japan and the Caribbean region. HTLV1, an RNA retrovirus, is a first cousin of the retrovirus responsible for acquired immunodeficiency syndrome (AIDS). Most of the other viruses under suspicion as cancer-causing fiends are DNA viruses, which probably integrate their dangerous genes directly into human DNA. RNA retroviruses, because they do not contain DNA, cannot infect cells by such a mechanism. You will recall from chapter 8 that DNA directs the formation of RNA. Normally this is one-way traffic from the nucleus to the cytoplasm. However, by an incredible trick of nature, the retroviruses can direct the reverse synthesis of DNA using RNA as a template by using a unique enzyme called reverse transcriptase. The newly formed DNA can then integrate into human DNA by the same mechanism the DNA viruses use.

Patients with AIDS have a high risk of developing two forms of cancer, Kaposi's sarcoma and malignant lymphoma. In AIDS it is likely that the onset of lymphoma is in some way related to the generalized disruption of the immune system. Like AIDS patients, transplant patients on long-term immunosuppression are also at increased risk for malignant lymphoma. Recently, a new herpeslike virus turned up in Kaposi tumor cells. Whether this is simply a viral passenger or in some way related to the development of the sarcoma is unknown. Although the relationship between viruses and human cancer is unclear, in many animals viruses have a definite causal role.

The geographic incidence of liver cancer (hepatocellular carcinoma) correlates strongly with the prevalence of chronic hepatitis B virus (HBV) infection. Chronic HBV infection causes a form of chronic inflammation of the liver that often ends up as cirrhosis and sometimes as liver cancer. In areas with a high HBV prevalence, such as Southeast Asia, Japan, and Central Africa, the incidence of liver cancer is 50 times greater than in the western world. In these high endemic areas, 80 percent to 90 percent of patients with liver cancer have livers infected with HBV. Recent studies also implicate the hepatitis C virus as a possible cause of liver cancer. Researchers accept that chronic ingestion of a food contaminant called aflatoxin is an important cause of some liver cancers. However, dietary intake of this chemical is common in those regions with a strong HBV prevalence, and whether aflatoxin is carcinogenic on its own or as a cofactor for HBV is still debated. Chronic viral infection of the liver cells by the hepatitis virus probably plays a significant role in the development of liver cancer (hepatocellular carcinoma) in such regions.

Many viruses consist largely of DNA. After entering the cell nucleus, the virus cleaves a portion of the host DNA and integrates its genetic material into the human DNA. As cells divide, the viral DNA transmits wrong signals that interfere with information coming from the human genes. The process is somewhat analogous to what happens when a "virus" contaminates computer programs. The program misreads the code. Over a period of time the program's mistakes accumulate and replicate, and eventually the computer malfunctions in some way. In the same way, the cell's program for growth and maturation fails because of rogue messages.

Viruses cause cancer in animals. They cause leukemia, lymphoma, and sarcomas in chickens, warty growths in cottontail rabbits, breast cancer in mice, and a variety of carcinomas and sarcomas in mice, rats, rabbits, and hamsters. A highly effective anticancer vaccine, developed against the chicken lymphoma virus in the early 1950s, successfully eradicated this economic hazard from poultry flocks.

No virus has yet proven itself to be unequivocally carcinogenic for humans. However, epidemiological studies have demonstrated very strong evidence of viral causation for some cancers. Papilloma viruses are DNA-containing viruses that have a particular affinity for the epithelium lining the surface of many organs, in particular squamous epithelium. In animals these viruses produce a variety of benign and malignant tumors. We find human papilloma viruses (HPV) in many human tumors, benign and malignant. However, the mere presence of a virus in cancer cells is no evidence of causation. We also find them occasionally in normal cells. Even if they are capable of causing cancer, how can we explain the fact that sometimes they appear to produce benign tumors rather than cancer?

Molecular biology techniques have cracked some papilloma secrets. Each papilloma virus has numerous genetic variants. Think of them as subspecies of a major species. Gradually we have an emerging picture of certain subtypes being strongly associated with certain cancers. The strongest association between HPV and any human cancer is with cancer of the cervix. The association is particularly compelling for subtypes 16 and 18. These HPV subtypes are present in many, but not all, low-grade dysplastic lesions of the cervix. Lesions harboring these variants are far more likely to progress to cancer than similar-appearing lesions without the virus. Lesions containing a different subtype are also less likely to progress. Despite its suspicious role in the development of cervical cancer, most authorities believe HPV is not the sole culprit. It is likely that on its own it does not drive dysplastic changes to full malignancy. It appears to have one or more allies lurking in its cellular neighborhood. These yet unidentified cofactors aid and abet the malignant process over a period of many years. One possible cofactor is another virus, the herpes simplex type 2 virus.

Epidemiologists found that early age of first sexual intercourse and multiple sexual partners put women in a high-risk category. They, and many gynecologists, postulate that cervical cancer is a sexually transmitted disease, caused primarily by HPV infection. Since some cervical cancers do not contain HPV, it seems unlikely that all cervical cancers are sexually transmitted. At the beginning of this chapter I mentioned that cancer was not a single disease and that it was inconceivable that all cancers would have the same cause. Keep this in mind when you read or hear about any cancer, such as cancer of the cervix. This also is probably not a single disease but a group of diseases with many overlapping similarities. Undoubtedly, it has more than one cause.

In some parts of the world, nonviral infections cause cancer. For example, infestation with the parasite Schistosoma causes bladder cancer in North Africa. In this condition the carcinogenic mechanism is probably long-standing chronic irritation and inflammation.

Diet may also influence cancer susceptibility. High fat intake may predispose to breast and colon cancer. On the other hand, generous fiber intake appears to protect against colon cancer. How does it protect us? The rapid transit time of food residue means less contact time with the lining of the colon. The most widely held theory is that if there are dietary carcinogens in the intestine in contact with the colonic mucosa, their threat is reduced by rapid elimination and less contact time.

In recent years molecular biologists have made tremendous progress in our understanding of the mechanisms and processes whereby normal cells change into malignant cells. However, apart from the few exceptions mentioned, we still have very little idea about what actually causes cancer. What is it that initiates the cancer process?

Hereditary Factors

For most cancers it is likely that a combination of hereditary susceptibility and some environmental agent in combination is the cause. For some cancers the environmental agent is more important, for others it is the hereditary factor. Some experts believe tobacco smoke is responsible for up to 30 percent of all cancers in the western world. Many would suggest that this figure is as high as 60 percent. Apart from lung cancer, it appears to play a causative role in cancer of the mouth, throat, larynx, esophagus, and bladder. The cancer risk associated with smoking depends primarily on the number of cigarettes smoked, which correlates closely with the duration of the habit. In comparison with nonsmokers, smokers are twice as likely to get bladder cancer and eight times as likely to get lung cancer. Approximately 90 percent of lung cancers occur in cigarette smokers and there is a strong correlation between the number of cigarettes smoked over a lifetime and the risk of developing lung cancer.

Virtually all doctors and scientists believe unreservedly that smoking causes cancer. Yet we all know friends or relatives who have smoked all their lives and who do not get cancer. Why is this? Obviously their cells are resistant to the onslaught of tobacco smoke. What makes these cells resistant is unknown. To add to the confusion, some nonsmokers get lung cancer. Furthermore, the types of lung cancer they get are similar to those caused by smoking. Are these individuals susceptible to some other unrecognized inhalant or it is that they are hypersensitive to tiny doses of tobacco smoke in their environment? Despite some evidence suggesting that such passive smoking may cause cancer in susceptible individuals, it is a rare phenomenon.

Clearly, hereditary genetic abnormalities are the cause of some cancers. Patients with the autosomal dominant familial Polyposis coli have thousands of tiny polyps scattered throughout their colons. Unless their colons are removed by preventive surgery, these patients develop colon cancer from the polyps at a young age. The abnormal gene responsible for this form of cancer has been identified and cloned. It is the APC (gene that is responsible for familial adenomatosis polyposis), and it is located on the long arm of chromosome 5. FAP is a rare condition and accounts for a minuscule number of colon cancers. It appears, then, that at one extreme hereditary genetic defects are all-important while at the other extreme environmental agents are the principal culprits. However, even environmental agents inflict their initial damage on our DNA.

Table 9.4 Cancers with a Known Hereditary Predisposition*

Tissue	Mutated Gene	Comment
Breast	BRCA1 BRCA2	Account for less than 10 percent of breast cancers
Colon	APC MSH2 & MLH1	Familial polyposis Coli (rare), also known as familial adenomatosis polyposis Hereditary nonpolyposis colon cancer Possibly 10 percent of all colon cancers
Eye	Rb	Retinoblastoma in children
Kidney	WTI VHL	Wilms' tumor in children von Hippel-Lindau syndrome Renal cell carcinoma
Nerves and soft tissue	NF1 p53	von Recklinhausen's syndrome Li-Fraumeni syndrome

**These are just a few of the cancers with known hereditary genetic mutations. Sometimes a mutated gene is responsible for more than one cancer type. For example, BRCA1 and BRCA2 mutations are also responsible for some familial ovarian cancers. Mutations in some of these genes (e.g., p53) also occurs after birth. These are acquired mutations.*

Most colon cancers are sporadic, i.e., they occur as isolated incidents with no apparent familial cause. However, apart from the cancer arising in FAP patients, there is one other form of familial colon cancer that arises in young adults. This condition is known as the hereditary nonpolyposis coli syndrome (also known as the Lynch syndrome). Such colon cancers are much commoner than previously suspected and comprise approximately 10 percent of all colon cancers. These patients frequently get multiple colonic cancers. Recently, the genetic abnormality causing this familial type of cancer has been identified as a mutation in a number of DNA mismatch-repair genes. These are located on chromosomes 2 and 5.

Retinoblastoma is a malignancy of the retinal cells in the eye. Loss of one of the growth suppressor genes called Rb, which resides on the long arm of chromosome 13, is the main mechanism responsible for this tumor. Patients with other specific hereditary diseases are also at increased risk for malignant tumors. Most patients with Von Recklinhausen's disease do not get cancer, but some do. Von Recklinhausen's disease is characterized by the presence of soft benign skin tumors called neurofibromas. These tumors arise from the cells lining the outer part of the nerves, and in 5 percent of patients one or more neurofibromas transform into sarcomas, usually after the disease has been present for many years. As in retinoblastoma, the mechanism underlying malignant transformation is loss of a suppressor gene. In this case the gene is on chromosome 17. Every gene in every nucleus has a partner, an allele, i.e., each cell has two or more copies (alleles) of each gene. If one is missing at birth because of a hereditary defect, its partner assumes some or all of its functions. However, if at a later date the second partner is deactivated, the gene loses its normal function. Such is the likely sequence of events in hereditary tumors caused by loss of suppressor genes. This is referred to as the "two-hit hypothesis." The first hit is hereditary and the cell functions normally until a second, acquired, hit deactivates the survivor.

The Li-Fraumeni syndrome is characterized by the development of multiple cancers in various tissues. Hereditary loss of suppressor p53 activity, due to multiple mutations, causes this syndrome.

Approximately 10 percent of breast cancers are familial. Mutations in two recently recognized genes, BRCA1 and BRCA2, are responsible for most of these. They are also responsible for many familial ovarian cancers.

Until recently no familial incidence of prostate cancer was recognized. New evidence suggests that a small number (probably less than 10 percent) of prostate cancers are hereditary. However, we know very little about the genes involved. No doubt, as interest in and research on this cancer increases, the damaging genes will reveal their secrets. As we learn more about cancer and genes, it is likely that we will find many more links between hereditary genetic defects and environmental carcinogens.

At the beginning of the chapter, I pointed out that cancer is not one disease and does not have one cause. Nevertheless, the mechanisms giving rise to the cancer processes of initiation and progression are similar for all cancers. DNA damage, whether hereditary or acquired, or some combination of both, is the underlying abnormality responsible for all cancers. One popular hypothesis on the causation of cancer is that many mutations arise daily. Our natural defense mechanisms repair most of these defects—but not all of them. The residual errors accumulate and in time trigger the onset of cancer.

Bibliography

Bartecchi, C.E., T.D. Mackenzie, and R.W. Schrier. The global tobacco epidemic. *Scientific American* 275, 5 (May 1995): 44–51.

_____. The human costs of tobacco use (1). *New England Journal of Medicine* 330, 13 (1994):907–12.

Bolin, T.D., R.H. Hunt, M.G. Korman, J.R. Lambert, A. Lee, and N.J. Talley. Helicobacter pylori and gastric neoplasia: Evolving concepts. *Medical Journal of Australia* 163, 5 (1995):253–55.

Davidson, N.E. Is hormone replacement therapy a risk? *Scientific American* 275 (1996):68.

Goldman, M. Cancer risk of low-level exposure. *Science* 271, 5257 (1996):1821–22.

Hanley, A.J., B.C. Choi, and E.J. Holowaty. Cancer mortality among Chinese migrants: A review. *International Journal of Epidemiology* 24, 2 (1995):255–65.

Kaiser, J. New data help toxicologists home in on assessing risks. *Science* 272, 5259 (1996):200.

Kase, L.M. Why community cancer clusters are often ignored. *Scientific American* 275 (1996):55–56.

Longnecker, M.P. Alcohol consumption and risk of cancer in humans: An overview. *Alcohol* 12, 2 (1995):87–96.

Lubin, J.H. Invited commentary: lung cancer and exposure to residential radon. *American Journal of Epidemiology* 140, 4 (1994):323–32.

Mackenzie, T.D., C.E. Bartecchi, and R.W. Schrier. The human costs of tobacco use. (2). *New England Journal of Medicine* 330, 14 (1994):975–80.

Majno, G., and I. Joris. *Cells, tissues, and disease: Principles of general pathology*, Cambridge, Mass.: Blackwell Science, 1996.

Masood, E. Cancer link to power cables 'exaggerated,' say critics. *Nature* 379, 6566 (1996):57.

Miller, E.C., and J.A. Miller. Milestones in chemical carcinogenesis. *Seminars in Oncology* 6, 4 (1979):445–60.

Mirvish, S.S. Role of N-nitroso compounds (NOC) and N-nitrosation in etiology of gastric, esophageal, nasopharyngeal and bladder cancer and contribution to cancer of known exposures to NOC. *Cancer Letters* 93, 1 (1995):17–48.

Mossman, B.T. Carcinogenesis and related cell and tissue responses to asbestos: A review. *Annals of Occupational Hygiene* 38, 4 (1994):617–24.

Reynolds, P., and E.T. Fontham. Passive smoking and lung cancer. *Annals of Medicine* 27, 6 (1995):633–40.

Roizman, B. New viral footprints in Kaposi's sarcoma. *New England Journal of Medicine* 332 (1995):1227–28.

Shopland, D.R. Tobacco use and its contribution to early cancer mortality with a special emphasis on cigarette smoking. *Environmental Health Perspectives* 103 (suppl. 8) (1995):131–42.

Willett, W.C., G.A. Coldtiz, and N.E. Mueller. Strategies for minimizing cancer risk. *Scientific American* 275: (1996):58–63.

Wynder, E.L., and J.E. Muscat. The changing epidemiology of smoking and lung cancer histology. *Environmental Health Perspectives* 103 (suppl. 8) (1995): 143–48.

CHAPTER 10

How Do Doctors Diagnose Cancer?

The road to diagnosis takes different paths, but it almost always ends at the pathologist's microscope. Some lump, symptom, or screen-detected abnormality takes the patient to a doctor's office. After the doctor's examination comes a series of laboratory tests and usually some X-rays and then a biopsy. The final diagnosis rests with the pathologist. Pathologists are physicians who specialize in laboratory medicine. Those who spend much of their time diagnosing cancer are surgical pathologists. Unlike the popular television autopsy detectives, they work to ensure that the living patient gets the most accurate diagnosis science can provide.

They scrutinize every millimeter of biopsied tissue, looking for minor or major cell abnormalities. They look for clues in the tumor's differentiation, in its mitoses, and in its growth pattern. They grade the abnormalities. They use other techniques, in particular immunohistochemistry, to solve difficult problems. Immunohistochemistry is a technique that uses special antibodies labeled with a color-coded detector to identify proteins and chemicals hidden in the cell. It often helps to identify the true nature of tumors that appear undifferentiated by ordinary microscopy. Accurate diagnosis and grading are important. They guide the surgeon or oncologist to the best treatment. They indicate what the future may hold.

The patients and the public may know little about surgical pathologists or their work—they are the "backroom boys and girls." However, within the hospital they make their presence felt in the clinics, on the wards, and at case conferences. Apart from issuing biopsy reports, they contribute in many ways to overall patient management. In addition to accurate diagnosis and grading, they provide accurate staging. For example, their reports on lymph node involvement (lymph node status) supply crucial staging information. Other tumor measurements in the pathology report, such as the identification of the oncogene HER2neu and estrogen or progesterone receptor status, also contribute important prognostic data.

Pathologists attend surgical, radiology, and oncology conferences to explain the nuances of unusual tumors. They advise on the adequacy of surgical margins and the need for surgical reexcision or radiotherapy. During surgery, they provide the surgeon with intraoperative consultations using a rapid diagnostic technique (frozen section diagnosis). In conjunction with radiologists and surgeons, they participate in "triple assessment" breast clinics. Here, difficult breast cancer problems are reviewed, discussed, and debated, in order to get the best team opinion, for individual patients. In many hospitals, pathologists perform fine needle aspiration biopsies, as well as reporting them. In oncology centers they take part in, and often run, the tumor board conferences. Many eminent pathologists in academic centers give expert opinions to other pathologists and clinicians around the world. Biopsy preparations on glass slides are small and can be sent anywhere by express mail. Some pathologists are considering the possibility of providing consultations on the Internet or by other telemedicine methods.

Cancer makes itself known to the patient in many ways. It may announce its arrival incidentally during a cancer screening program, or it may be picked up on an X-ray during investigation for some unconnected complaint. Sometimes a lump is found at a routine checkup. Under these circumstances the patient has no symptoms related to the cancer and often feels in perfect health. News that the detected abnormality might be cancer strikes like a thunderbolt. Further diagnostic tests follow to confirm the diagnosis. Usually, cancers detected in this manner are small and curable. Examples include carcinoma in situ of the cervix detected during a routine gynecological checkup or a small breast cancer detected by screening mammography.

If a lump on an outer surface, such as the back of a hand or the face, reaches a couple of millimeters in size we can see and feel it. Unfortunately, most lethal cancers grow deep beneath the body surface, e.g., in the breast, or within internal organs such as lungs, intestine, prostate, or kidneys and are symptomless until they have reached a few centimeters in size. By the time a tumor has reached the size of a grape it has probably been growing for two to nine years and contains approximately a billion cells. We find them at this stage because we have symptoms. Deep-seated tumors are detected by various radiologic imaging techniques such as X-rays and CT or MRI scans. Computerized tomography (CT) is a sophisticated form of X-ray that visualizes changes deep within the body. The magnetic resonance imaging (MRI) scan is a computerized image of magnetic signals coming from tissues. In some circumstances, the MRI scan gives a better image and more useful information than the CT scan does.

If we can find and diagnose small, early cancers we stand a great chance of curing them. At some stage in their evolution cancers learn to spread throughout the body, via lymphatics and bloodstream—they metastasize. Rarely can they do so while they are still only a few millimeters in size, usually they need to reach a few centimeters before metastasizing. Unfortunately, at the time of diagnosis, we often do not know when a tumor has reached this critical point.

In clinical practice how do you find precancers? In a number of situations it is easy. Good examples are skin cancer, cancer of the cervix (the outer portion of the womb or uterus), and breast cancer. We can identify malignant melanoma, a lethal form of skin cancer, in its earliest preinvasive phase. Any benign mole that increases in size, changes its color, or starts to bleed is suspicious, as is a new patch of irregular dark pigmentation anywhere on the skin. The diagnosis of early melanoma is confirmed by biopsy (removal of a small amount of tissue for microscopic analysis). Doctors identify other forms of less serious skin cancer (squamous and basal cell carcinomas) because they present as visible persistent slightly scaly patches, plaques or lumps, usually on the sun-exposed skin of the middle-aged and elderly. All forms of early skin cancer can be cured by local excision.

A gynecologist can sample cells from the cervix. It is not so easy to look at cells from the brain, from bone, or from deep within the pancreas. Furthermore, even if you could sample these organs, you would not know where to take the sample from. The gynecologist takes cells from an entire area of cervix that is prone to malignancy.

Dysplasia and carcinoma in situ of the cervix (commonly called CIN, or cervical intraepithelial neoplasia) are diagnosed by gently rubbing the surface of the cervix with a spatula and transferring the abnormal exfoliated cells to a glass slide. Because tumor cells stick poorly to each other, they shed more easily than normal cells do and thousands of cells are removed easily with a spatula. After microscopic diagnosis, the precancerous surface is removed by relatively minor surgery or by laser destruction.

Ductal carcinoma in situ (DCIS) is the earliest recognizable form of breast cancer. The female breast consists of connective tissue, fat, and a branching system of canals lined by epithelial cells. These canals or ducts are encased by basement membrane. As carcinoma cells accumulate and fill the ducts, small deposits of calcium precipitate within debris and around dead tumor cells. Because it is resistant to X-ray penetration, calcium lights up in a special breast X-ray known as a mammogram. This highlights the DCIS. A small biopsy or needle aspiration from the mammographic abnormality provides sufficient tissue for pathology. For most DCIS patients, a lumpectomy or segmentectomy (surgical removal of a segment of breast), sometimes followed by local radiotherapy to the breast, is curative. Local removal may be inadequate for those rare cases where DCIS is scattered throughout much of the breast. These patients usually require a mastectomy (removal of the entire breast). While the idea of losing a breast is frightening, the patient can be assured that a subsequent invasive cancer is thus prevented and that she will not die from DCIS.

Some treatable conditions show premalignant dysplasia: long-standing skin ulcers, some skin moles, the mucosa lining the mouth in heavy cigarette smokers, some stomach ulcers, the inflamed lining of the lower esophagus where it enters the stomach (this is called Barrett's esophagus), the lining of the womb in some postmenopausal women with hormonal imbalances, and the colon in patients suffering from long-standing and extensive ulcerative colitis. Surgical removal of dysplastic tissue prevents cancer.

Surgery also cures other precancers. Intestinal polyps, the precursors of colon cancer, can be removed through an endoscope (a sort of flexible telescope for looking at the inside of hollow organs such as esophagus, stomach, intestine, or bladder). Intestinal polyps usually afflict the middle-aged and elderly. Many patients have more than one polyp—often a dozen or even more. A rare form of intestinal polyps called familial adenomatosis polyposis (FAP), characterized by the presence of thousands of colonic polyps, is a more serious condition. This hereditary disease, affecting 1 in 5,000 individuals, inevitably ends in cancer unless the colon is removed. In patients with FAP, the progression of polyps to cancer is prevented by colectomy.

Cytologists and pathologists recognize dysplasia as the earliest form of premalignancy, and the diagnostic tool they use is the microscope. In the future they will look for earlier DNA abnormalities using molecular biological techniques. Even more useful will be the ability to detect the agents causing cancer, when these are recognizable. Already the human papilloma virus (HPV) is the object of intense research in cervical cancer screening. Since there is strong evidence that HPV causes many or most cervical cancers, researchers are hopeful that its detection in cervical tissue will prove useful as a screening procedure.

Unfortunately, most cancers are not diagnosed at a very early stage or in their premalignant phase. Often, some symptom announces the beginning of a long and frightening battle. What this symptom is depends on where the cancer is and the size of the tumor. Sometimes a lump or sore is so slow-growing that the patient thinks it is something trivial and delays seeking medical attention. Such tumors are commonly present for years before the patient goes to the doctor. If a lump is located anywhere near the body surface, such as breast, chest wall, axilla (armpit), groin, or neck, the patient will probably feel it. Sometimes, a friend or relative may be the first to notice it. It is important to realize that not all lumps are malignant; in fact, most are benign and innocuous, and some are not even tumors. Some lumps are cysts or inflamed tissue.

Cancers are not painful or tender; they contain no nerves. However, if they damage or destroy surrounding tissue (a frequent occurrence) or infiltrate nerves, they may be painful. For example, cancer of the stomach may cause pain and symptoms like those of a peptic ulcer from ulceration of the mucosal lining. With tumors of the intestine that are large enough to cause obstruction, the patient will have crampy abdominal pain. More often, intestinal tumors produce anemia from chronic blood loss and are otherwise asymptomatic.

Tumors involving bone, whether primary sarcomas or metastatic carcinomas, are often painful. Tiny fractures in the bone surrounding the tumor cause the pain. Commonly the pain follows some minor exertion or trivial injury. Symptoms due to metastatic tumor sometimes precede symptoms from the primary tumor.

Sadly, most internal cancers are asymptomatic until they have reached a large size. Even at this stage most symptoms, such as weight loss, general fatigue, or loss of appetite are nonspecific, and the diagnosis may be delayed or even missed until too late. Some cancers are first diagnosed at autopsy.

Rarely, a small occult cancer manifests itself by producing some form of paraneoplastic syndrome. These syndromes are due to the inappropriate production and release of a hormone or hormonelike chemical. As a result the patient may complain of any one of a wide variety of apparently unrelated symptoms—muscle weakness, a sensation of pins and needles in the fingers and toes, dark velvety skin patches in the armpits, skin itch without a rash, obesity or wasting, and a variety of other symptoms that depend on what type of hormone the tumor produces. (See the discussion of lung cancer in chapter 6.)

Many benign diseases share the same symptoms as cancer. Brain cancer may cause headache. Headache is a common, usually trivial, symptom and usually has no associated organic disease. It assumes more significance if it is persistent or severe or associated with some other symptoms such as vomiting, speech difficulty, blurred vision, or weakness of an arm or leg. Benign brain tumors such as meningiomas or neuromas may produce the same set of symptoms as brain cancer, because they compress normal brain structures. Benign gastric ulcers are common. They produce abdominal pain and the patient is often anemic from slow blood loss into the intestine over a period of months. Cancer of the stomach can produce identical symptoms. Tuberculosis produces a chronic cough; sometimes sputum (spittle) is blood-tinged. Lung cancer produces the same symptoms. Benign enlargement of the prostate is common in elderly males and causes difficulty in passing urine; so does prostate cancer.

How then does a doctor distinguish benign from malignant conditions in each of these situations? At the initial interview it is unlikely that the family doctor will be able to diagnose cancer with any degree of confidence. In many situations, he or she may be able to reassure the patient that all is well. A young woman in her early twenties worries about a breast lump. She has been bombarded with stories about breast cancer in newspapers and women's magazines, and now she is terrified that she too might have cancer. On physical examination, the physician notes that the lump is about 1cm, is freely mobile within the breast, and not tethered to surrounding tissue. The remainder of the breast is normal, as is the axilla. The patient has no other symptoms, appears to be in perfect health, and has no family history of breast cancer. Based on the combination of these positive and negative findings and the knowledge that breast cancer is vanishingly rare in this age group, the physician confidently diagnoses a fibroadenoma and reassures her that this is a benign tumor that will not change into cancer. If she wishes to have it removed, for peace of mind, this can be done by a minor surgical procedure. There will be no significant cosmetic defect and the pathologist will confirm the diagnosis. This case is easy.

However, suppose a patient has the same apparent lump and is in her thirties and her mother had died of breast cancer at the age of forty. Despite the lump's apparent benign physical appearance, the physician will be less confident of the diagnosis and will insist or strongly advise that the lump be removed for microscopic diagnosis. In this situation the strong family history of breast cancer assumes greater importance than the physical examination.

Like most professionals in all walks of life, a physician bases a decision on expertise, experience, knowledge, and circumstances. Often a symptom or set of circumstances alerts the physician to the possibility that the patient may have cancer. At this stage he or she needs more information before making a definitive diagnosis. The physician gets this information by a variety of methods—by various laboratory or radiology tests, or possibly by getting a second opinion from an expert who specializes in the area under suspicion. A 58-year-old woman has not had a menstrual period since the age of 45. Now she has started menstruating again or so she thinks. The light bleeding has been present on and off for the past two months, not at all like it used to be before her periods stopped. Her physician knows that one of the commonest causes of postmenopausal bleeding is cancer of the endometrium (the epithelial lining of the womb) and refers her urgently to a gynecologist, who curettes a sample of tissue from the uterus. A surgical pathologist confirms that it is endometrial cancer. A few days later the gynecologist carries out a hysterectomy. The pathologist finds that the cancer is well differentiated, low grade, and confined to the inner wall of the uterus. This is an early-stage tumor. These pathological findings are highly favorable and indicate an excellent prognosis. The patient is cured by early surgery and requires no chemotherapy or radiotherapy. Another straightforward case.

The art of diagnosis begins with a good interview, during which the doctor takes a careful history of the complaint. How long has the symptom been present? Has anything changed in the recent past? Are there other symptoms? After some probing questions, the doctor builds in his or her mind a picture (at this stage an incomplete and sometimes vague picture) of what is going on and considers the possible diseases that might cause the symptom or set of symptoms. The next step is a physical examination. If a lump is present, where is it? What size is it? Is it soft or hard? Does it move easily, or is it fixed to surrounding tissues? Is there any evidence that the "lump" has spread to draining lymph nodes or to the liver? Are the lymph nodes or liver enlarged?

Armed with this information and taking into consideration the patient's age, sex, past history, family history, and possibly occupational history, the doctor modifies the mental picture and shortens the list of diagnostic possibilities. This list is known as the differential diagnosis. From the theoretical and textbook point of view, the differential diagnosis may include twenty or more possibilities. In practice, experience and statistical probability suggest that the physician needs to consider only two or three diagnoses.

The next step is to narrow the possible suspects to the one most likely diagnosis. A few laboratory tests or X-rays may do this. A 60-year-old man presents with recent back pain. On questioning, he states that he also has some difficulty passing urine and that this has been present for more than a year. He has no relevant past or family history. Physical examination reveals a firm to hard prostate gland, and the doctor suspects that the patient has cancer of the prostate gland, with metastases to the vertebral bones. The physician suspects this because (1) cancer of the prostate is common in this age group, (2) cancer is the commonest disease to cause a firm or hard prostate, and (3) prostate cancer frequently spreads to the lower spine. An alternative possibility is that the patient has two coincidental and unrelated abnormalities. Degeneration of the disk between the vertebral bones frequently causes low back pain, as does arthritis. Benign prostatic enlargement is common (almost universal) in this age group and sometimes it has a firm consistency.

A blood test in the local hospital laboratory shows an elevated prostate specific antigen (PSA) level, and X-rays show irregular mottled bones in the spine, consistent with metastatic cancer. These abnormalities confirm the diagnosis of prostate cancer—almost. One last procedure, a prostatic needle biopsy, carried out by a urologist, gives the final and definitive diagnosis. As illustrated in this case, the final step is to confirm the diagnostic suspicion of cancer by examining a piece of tissue microscopically. Although it is often not necessary to perform a biopsy to confirm a benign process, it is only in rare and exceptional circumstances that doctors will treat a patient for cancer without a tissue diagnosis. The diagnostic process flows from a detailed history of symptoms, through physical examination, to preliminary X-rays and laboratory tests, and finally to pathological examination.

There are often variations in the process. If the suspicious lesion is in the skin, then the quickest way to get a diagnosis is to just biopsy the skin and forget about intermediate superfluous tests. If the skin lesion is small, the doctor can do an excision biopsy. This removes and treats the suspicious area as well as providing tissue for diagnosis. Sometimes, X-rays or laboratory tests give inconclusive results and need to be followed by additional laboratory or X-ray procedures. The initial X-ray image may not be abnormal enough to give an answer; subsequent CT (computerized tomography) or MRI (magnetic resonance image) may be spectacularly more informative.

Sometimes it is difficult to make a definitive diagnosis. There are times when even a tissue sample may not yield the diagnosis, at least not initially. A 58-year-old man has vague abdominal pain and discomfort. He has a long history of alcohol abuse. After a variety of inconclusive tests, a CT (computerized tomography) scan shows a large mass, deep within the upper abdomen, in the relatively inaccessible region of his pancreas. This is strongly suspicious for malignancy. As always, final proof of cancer rests on identifying cancer cells microscopically. If the patient has cancer, major surgery with all its potential implications is indicated. If he has pancreatitis, then rest, time, and minor medications are prescribed. To examine pancreatic cells for malignancy, a radiologist inserts a very fine needle into the abdominal mass and aspirates fluid and cells. Some irregular atypical cells, suspicious for malignancy, are identified. Although the microscopic findings are very abnormal, the pathologist is unwilling to make a definitive diagnosis of malignancy. Possibly, the abnormal cell appearance is caused by something other than cancer, a common enough occurrence. Eventually, after much discussion and consultation between patient and physician, and between physician, surgeon, radiologist, and pathologist, a small piece of tissue is removed from the pancreas by biopsy during a laparotomy (surgical exploration of the abdomen). This shows that the abnormal mass is due to chronic pancreatitis with prominent scar tissue, the result of heavy alcohol consumption over many years. The suspicious cells seen on the microscope were rapidly regenerating cells attempting to replace damaged or dead tissue, and in this situation simulated closely the changes seen in cancer. A false positive diagnosis of malignancy could have had disastrous consequences for all concerned. The patient would have had unnecessary, possibly life-threatening, surgery. The hospital and all physicians concerned with the case could have found themselves at the wrong end of a large malpractice suit. Most cancers can be diagnosed readily. Occasionally a definitive diagnosis cannot be made at the first presentation because the evidence is insufficient. In such cases close follow-up and repeat biopsy may be necessary later.

Newer radiology and laboratory techniques are improving diagnoses in difficult cases. Radiologists, physicists, and computer programmers are developing new diagnostic imaging techniques to enhance the resolution of tiny X-ray abnormalities. The University of Chicago School of Medicine uses computerized image analysis and neural network artificial intelligence programs to diagnose subtle mammographic shadows. This sophisticated technology often picks up early abnormalities missed by humans. It is possible that in the future similar programs will examine a large number of screening mammograms. Similar technology is finding a place in screening cytology. Microscopic screening for early dysplasia in cervical cytology specimens is labor-intensive, time-consuming and tedious. Furthermore, the diagnosis depends on variable human factors. Well-trained cytologists on their best days are highly reliable in picking up mild abnormalities. Under less than ideal conditions cytologists can miss not just subtle changes but even more advanced life-threatening abnormalities. A few abnormal cells often lie hidden between, and surrounded by, thousands of normal cells. A tired cytologist can easily overlook such cells. Image analysis combined with artificial intelligence computer programs take the tedium out of cytology screening; it is accurate and rapid. This technology has already found its way into a number of larger laboratories, and undoubtedly in the near future it will find widespread acceptance.

Molecular biology research techniques, in particular the polymerase chain reaction (PCR), are gradually finding diagnostic oncological applications in clinical laboratories. PCR techniques amplify minuscule bits of DNA, suitable for mutation analysis of what are called gene rearrangements. Gene rearrangements often act as marker abnormalities for specific cancers. Pathologists commonly face the diagnostic problem of distinguishing certain types of benign but atypical lymphoid hyperplasia from malignant lymphoma. Molecular biology techniques applied to biopsied tissue can distinguish between a monoclonal proliferation (cancer) and benign polyclonal hyperplasia. The same techniques can identify micrometastases in bone marrow samples used in clinical staging. PCR is so sensitive that it can pluck out one malignant cell hidden amidst 100,000 normal cells. PCR and other molecular techniques may soon help oncologists select the most appropriate chemotherapeutic regime for a particular cancer. For example, it is now possible to check whether a tumor has an activated gene for multidrug resistance or whether it has a mutated version of p53. Such information may help select the best drug for a particular patient's cancer.

The combined efforts of biologists, biochemists, physicists, and computer experts ensure that today's research techniques will form the basis for tomorrow's routine diagnostic tests.

Bibliography

Buckman, R. *What you really need to know about cancer.* London: Macmillan, 1996.

Giger, M.L., and Pelizzari, C.A.. Advances in tumor imaging. *Scientific American* 275 (1996):76–78.

Hanks, G.E., and P.T. Scardino. Does screening for prostate cancer make sense? *Scientific American* 275 (1996):80–81.

Maranto, G. Should women in their 40s have mammograms? *Scientific American* 275 (1996):79.

Naber, S.P. Molecular pathology—Detection of neoplasia. *New England Journal of Medicine* 331, 22 (1994):1508–10.

Putterman, C. and E. Ben Chetrit. Clinical problem solving. Testing, testing, testing.... *New England Journal of Medicine* 333, 18 (1995):1208–11.

Sidransky, D. Advances in cancer detection. *Scientific American* 275 (1996):70–75.

CHAPTER 11

Treatment Principles and Strategies

In many patients' minds, cancer treatment equals nausea, vomiting, loss of hair, and just about the worst imaginable hangover. For most patients, therapy is nowhere near as terrible as this.

There are three standard approaches to curative cancer treatment. In addition, the last fifteen years have spawned a number of new innovative treatments, some highly successful and many still experimental. Patients gone beyond the curative stage have a wide range of palliative treatments available.

Surgery

Surgery is most successful for slow-growing cancers, and for localized disease it is often curative. This is the standard and only form of treatment required for many cancers. Skin cancers and numerous other cancers such as those involving the thyroid, salivary glands, stomach, or intestine are treated primarily by surgery. The rationale behind curative surgery is to remove the entire malignancy before it has spread. This means excision of the tumor and a margin of surrounding normal tissue. The amount of tissue removed depends on the type of tumor and its anatomic location. In addition, the surgeon often removes the adjacent lymph nodes, provided no serious disfigurement or complications will follow.

A typical example is colon cancer. The surgeon removes the tumor, with a length of intestine on either side of the tumor, and draining lymph nodes are removed with this type of surgery. With other types of cancer, such as breast cancer, the lymph nodes are often just sampled. Those who favor sampling a few axillary (armpit) lymph nodes, rather than removing them all, argue that the real purpose of removing these nodes is to get an accurate tumor stage, and sampling is adequate for this purpose. Furthermore, they argue that the complication rate after radical axillary node dissection is often unjustifiably high. The main complication is lymphodema, a distressing permanent swelling of the arm due to poor lymph drainage.

Surgical techniques, particularly reconstructive surgery combined with plastic surgery, have improved immensely over the past twenty years. The newer techniques enhance the patient's life-style and improve the quality of life. In the past, limb amputation was the only treatment for patients with bone cancer in an arm or leg. Now orthopedic surgeons perform limb-sparing surgery for many such patients. They remove the tumor-bearing bone and surrounding normal bone and insert a metal prosthesis as they would for, say, a hip replacement. Often they also need to replace an adjacent joint, usually the knee. Bone cancers treatable through such techniques frequently arise in children, and limb-sparing surgery allows them to retain excellent function. As the child grows, the surgeon elongates the prosthesis to keep up with growth. Even more impressive than the above surgery is a new limb-lengthening technique (which is also used to help a child with a congenitally short leg). The technique can be used for all bone tumors except those too near a joint. The surgeon excises the tumor and an adjacent segment of normal bone, for example, in the shin. He or she then places a tubular sleeve of periosteum, stripped from normal bone, in the gap left behind. The periosteum is the membrane lining the outer bone surface, and it lays down new bone. Slowly, millimeter by millimeter, new bone fills in the gap left by the excised bone. That is, the patient grows a new bone segment. After about a year or eighteen months, the gap fills in completely. In the meantime, an orthopedic external frame stabilizes the leg. This miraculous surgery allows the patient to grow a new segment of an arm or leg.

Sometimes it is not possible to remove a cancer completely. However, the surgeon may remove more than 90 percent of the tumor and restore good function to the organ affected. Sometimes it is possible to kill the residual tumor with radiotherapy. One of the critical shortcomings of surgery is that tiny, microscopic, fingerlike extensions from the cancer may spread beyond the filed of surgery. These foci, unseen by the surgeon, are left behind. Likewise, tiny metastases may have spread to lymph nodes or other tissues beyond the margins of the surgical excision.

The pathologist's report, indicating the tumor type, its grade, and how close it is to surgical margins helps the surgeon or oncologist predict with considerable accuracy whether the tumor is likely to have spread beyond the surgical resection. For example, since basal cell carcinomas of the skin almost never metastasize, chemotherapy is pointless. Likewise, although malignant melanoma is an aggressive killer, if the pathologist's report indicates an invasive thickness of 0.76mm or less, it rarely metastasizes. In contrast, if the excised tumor is high-grade non-Hodgkin's lymphoma, the clinician knows that irrespective of surgical margins the tumor has probably spread already to other tissues, and chemotherapy will benefit the patient. In fact, it will cure most patients even if it has already spread widely, as lymphoma cells are very sensitive to chemotherapy. In this situation, tumor type and grade are more important than stage.

Radiation Therapy

For some cancers, radiation therapy is more suitable than surgery and just as effective. In some centers, up to 60 percent of all patients with cancer are treated with radiation therapy sometime during the course of their illness. The radiotherapy may be administered on its own or combined with surgery or chemotherapy. Like surgery, radiotherapy is a local treatment. It kills only cells within the radiation field. Some tumors are highly radiosensitive, such as testicular cancers, Hodgkin's disease, and some low-grade non-Hodgkin's lymphomas. Others, such as most soft tissue sarcomas, are highly radioresistant. Radiotherapy uses high-energy ionizing radiation, which damages one or both strands of the DNA molecule in tumor cells. This prevents them from dividing and growing. Normal cells nearby are also damaged. However, normal cells can repair DNA damage more rapidly than cancer cells. This is the reason why radiation is usually delivered in small fractionated doses whose size is altered over a period of five or six weeks. After each dose, normal tissue recovers quickly, whereas the effects of the fractionated doses are cumulative to the cancer DNA. Radiation can be delivered by external beam radiation, by implanting radioactive seeds into the tumor, or by administering radioactive isotopes.

External radiation is the commonest, and the kind of machine used to deliver the lethal beams depends on the type and extent of the tumor. Advanced technology allows the radiation beam to be concentrated on the tumor while causing little damage to surrounding normal tissues. Special X-ray computer programs called simulators allow the radiation oncologist to visualize a map of the tumor outline and to calculate and modify the dose delivered to each area on the map.

Radioactive seeds, needles, or capsules implanted directly into the tumor sometimes help. This type of radiation therapy is called brachytherapy. For some cancers brachytherapy is more suitable than external beam radiation.

Radioactive isotopes are not used very often. The classic example is in the treatment of some thyroid cancers. The thyroid gland concentrates iodine in its cells; it requires iodine to make the hormone thyroxine. Some thyroid cancers retain the ability to take up and concentrate iodine, including radioactive iodine (I^{131}). The radioactive iodine molecule taken up by the malignant thyroid cells destroys them. Even after they have metastasized, some thyroid cancers continue to take up and concentrate iodine and they can be treated with radioactive iodine. Because treatment with radioactive iodine damages normal thyroid cells as well, it is necessary to give the patient replacement thyroxine hormone, which is simply taken as a tablet every day.

Advances in radiobiology (the study of how cells and tissue are affected by radiation) allied to new physics technology and computer science are paying dividends for cancer patients. Radiotherapists are researching new ways to increase the radiosensitivity of tumor cells and at the same time increase radioresistance in normal cells. For example, oxygen and certain drugs increase tumor sensitivity and numerous research programs are exploring ways to treat oxygen-starved tumor cells to kill them more easily. Physicists are designing more powerful radiation-producing machines. Computer scientists strive to find ways to keep the deadly beams within the confines of the tumor. In the treatment referred to as conformal radiotherapy, the radiation beams conform closely to the shape of the tumor, and radiation therapists can change the shape and direction of the beam as the tumor changes shape and size. Conformal radiotherapy is particularly useful for tumors in poorly accessible areas such as the prostate. Like other branches of medicine, radiation therapy is advancing at a great pace.

Sometimes tumors are extremely radiosensitive; the malignant cells are killed easily by radiation beams (X-rays). A classic example of where radiotherapy is curative is cancer of the testis. The commonest type of testicular cancer is seminoma, a malignant tumor of the sperm-forming cells. These tumors occur in young men and spread to the lymph nodes in the back of the abdomen—the retroperitoneal lymph nodes. While a surgeon can easily remove a testicular tumor, dissection of the retroperitoneal nodes is very difficult. In the past, radiation to the retroperitoneal lymph nodes produced dramatic cures in a very high percentage of patients whose metastases were confined to the lymph nodes. Nowadays patients are treated mostly by surgery for the testicular tumor and chemotherapy, since chemotherapy destroys cancer cells that have spread beyond the lymph nodes.

Like surgery, radiation therapy is effective only locally. The radiation must be directed at the anatomic location of the tumor. Neither surgery nor radiation treatment can address the problem of tumor cells that break away from the main tumor mass and lodge at distant, unknown sites. For these cases, chemotherapy provides the best chance of cure.

Chemotherapy

Chemotherapy has the advantage that is permeates the entire body and destroys malignant cells lurking silently in the lungs, liver, bone, and elsewhere. This, at least, is the desired effect. The action can be likened to the effect of antibiotics on bacteria. Antibiotics get into the bloodstream and eventually surround and destroy the bacteria no matter where they hide. The problem with chemotherapy is that it wipes out normal cells also. Oncologists and pharmacologists over the past couple of decades have struggled to identify drugs that are toxic to tumor cells and safe for normal cells. The ideal chemotherapy cocktails hit DNA and the enzymes and proteins of the dividing malignant cells while sparing normal cells. The balance between targeting cancer cells and preserving normal cells is a delicate one that is not always achieved. Some cancer cells become resistant to chemotherapeutic drugs by various devious, almost intelligent mechanisms. Cells contain specific genes that switch on tiny cell-membrane pumps to remove certain chemicals from the cell, and cancer cells are no exception. In adapting to the chemotherapy, these genes can jump to life and remove chemotherapy drugs from the cells.

Imagine a small garden with beautiful shrubs and flowers, some of them growing in a handsome rock garden. One day, to your horror, you look in and find thousands of tiny insects eating the leaves. As you look more closely, you notice that they have spread over the entire garden. Out comes the insecticide, which you spray unsparingly over the entire garden. The nasty insects scurry beneath the pebbles and shrubs. Within a few hours they are all dead, or so you think. Next day, you find that a few dozen of the critters have survived and are as hungry as ever. You spray them again, this time with no obvious effect. The survivors, somehow or other, are resistant to the insecticide. You buy a different spray, and another, and another. They are no use. At this stage, the few survivors have multiplied and there are hundreds of insects ravaging your garden.

So too with resistant cancer cells and chemotherapy. Somewhat like an accelerated evolutionary process, while sensitive tumor cells are dying all around them, drug-resistant cells multiply unharmed as their membranes pump the man-made poisons out of their cytoplasm and back into the circulation. Multidrug resistance is a major obstacle to successful chemotherapy for many patients.

With some cancers, chemotherapy can kill the entire population of tumor cells and cure the patient. With others, it can kill almost the entire population. The few remaining cells may be too damaged to grow again; this patient is also cured. However, with some cancers, the few chemoresistant surviving cells grow and spread after a variable dormant period, often years. Finally, and unfortunately, some cancers are highly resistant from the beginning.

Doctors measure treatment success in terms of "five-year survival." They know that up to five years is needed to see whether therapy has been successful. In reality, even five-year survival cannot always be equated with cure. A small number of cancers will grow back after the magic five-year period. We now know that some cancer metastases remain dormant for periods of ten years or even longer and then recur. How do doctors know which type of treatment is best for an individual patient? Proper treatment is based on a combination of (1) tumor type and stage, (2) the patient's physical circumstances, such as age, pregnancy, allergies, and general overall medical condition (good kidney, liver, and heart function, for example), and (3) whether the purpose of treatment is cure, prolonged survival or pure palliation. In the past, doctors selected treatment according to what their teachers told them and on their expertise, intuition, and common sense. Often treatment was based on anecdote or unproven opinion. Many treatments were ineffective or toxic. Examples include gastric freezing for peptic ulcers (useless), radiation therapy for acne or enlarged thymuses (caused thyroid cancer), and thalidomide for sedation during pregnancy. Nowadays, cancer specialists also have the benefit of clinical trials.

Doctors realize that what appears like the best treatment, from an intuitive or common-sense point of view, is sometimes wrong. Clinical trials examine scientifically what is the best treatment for a particular cancer. They take into account all known prognostic factors. A large number of patients from multiple centers, often from major cancer centers in many different countries, are entered into the study. The results of treatment A are then compared to treatment B for efficacy, acceptability, and complications. The researchers publish the results in reputable, peer-reviewed, international medical journals and this information is disseminated to cancer specialists around the world. Journal editors comment on, applaud, or criticize the way the trial was performed. If they find flaws or omissions in the study, they let their readers know. Such clinical trials help the patient and the doctor to select the best proven treatment. Clinical trials are often run as double-blind trials in which neither the patient nor the doctor knows which drugs are given to which patients. An independent research agency analyzes the results. In this way statistical bias is eliminated. Clinical trials involve important ethical issues. Patients must understand how the trials are constructed and organized. They must understand that they have no obligation to participate in such trials. After receiving full and proper explanation, they give informed consent. Every safeguard possible must be made to ensure that the trials include only those patients for whom no better treatment is known. The results of trials are continuously monitored, and if any serious harmful effect is detected, the trial is terminated. In general, patients in trials benefit, as they have an opportunity to take advantage of the newest and possibly the best treatments available.

New drugs, less toxic and more specific for individual cancers with more specific activity against the various components of the cell cycle, are continually being developed. The anticancer pharmaceutical industry is a multibillion-dollar industry. The massive development in biotechnology has also spawned new and innovative treatments.

Other than anticancer medication, a wide variety of drugs play a crucial supportive role for the cancer patient—antibiotics, antinausea drugs, and analgesics (painkillers). Chemotherapy often kills normal rapidly proliferating cells such as bone marrow and immune cells, leaving patients susceptible to infection. In addition to common bacterial infections, immunosuppressed patients are prone to get unusual viral and fungal infections. New bone-marrow-stimulating drugs are particularly helpful in preventing infection in these patients.

Sometimes therapeutic decisions are difficult, as illustrated in the following case history. A 32-year-old woman, after eight years of heartbreaking infertility, was at last pregnant. Her intense joy was shattered when an ultrasound scan showed that she had cancer of the ovary. Surgery and pathology confirmed this. The ray of good news was that the tumor was a dysgerminoma; this is a highly chemosensitive cancer. She required life-saving chemotherapy. The dilemmas facing herself, her husband, her obstetrician, and her oncologist included major moral, ethical, and religious issues, along with the medical problems. The easiest, most straightforward medical decision would have been immediate termination of pregnancy, followed by a regime of chemotherapy standard for this particular tumor. The patient and her husband rejected this option. After a comprehensive computer-assisted search, and a study of the medical literature for reports on similar cases, the doctors offered a compromise solution. The fetus was allowed to develop to a stage where all fetal tissues were formed before instituting chemotherapy. Treatment began at twenty weeks of pregnancy. A normal baby girl was delivered on time. The mother is cured and her 5-year-old daughter has developed normally and shows no side effects of the intrauterine chemical assault.

Bone Marrow and Stem Cell Transplantation

For patients with certain forms of leukemia and lymphoma, another type of treatment is available, namely, bone marrow transplantation (BMT). Some leukemias have a high relapse rate or respond poorly to chemotherapy, and for patients with these cancers BMT is often a lifesaver. The doctors take normal bone marrow from the patient while he or she is in remission and store it, until required, in liquid nitrogen. The hematologists or oncologists use intensive chemotherapy to destroy any recurrent tumor in the marrow. This also destroys the normal marrow and leaves the patient unable to fight off even the most trivial infection. The stored normal marrow, given to the patient through an intravenous infusion, fortunately returns to the bone-marrow cavity on its own and grows quickly to produce infection-fighting white blood cells. During the time between marrow destruction and recovery, the patient is nursed in a germ-free environment and can have white blood cell transfusions to tide him or her over the critical period, if this is required. The medical term used for this type of BMT, whereby the patient is his or her own donor, is autologous BMT.

Sometimes autologous BMT is not possible because the patient has no period of complete remission. Taken from such a patient, tumor cells might recontaminate the bone marrow. The way around this problem is to use marrow from someone else. This is termed an allogenic transplant. The donor should be someone, usually a family member, with a close match for certain transplantation immune genes. Unlike the autologous patients, allogenic patients occasionally have additional problems. Because their BMT is foreign tissue, they run the risk that their bodies will reject the marrow. Alternatively, the foreign marrow thinks the host, i.e., the patient, is foreign, and launches an all-out war to reject host tissue. This is known as graft-versus-host disease. Fortunately, it can be treated.

Many countries have bone-marrow transplantation programs. In the United States, the National Marrow Donor Program (NMDP) keeps a computerized database of possible donors.

A new alternative to autologous BMT is peripheral blood stem cell transplantation. Bone marrow cells grow from special precursor cells in the marrow, called stem cells. Stem cells divide and differentiate into the precursors of white blood cells, red blood cells, and platelets. A small number make their way into the peripheral blood and, in the company of other blood cells, circulate throughout the body. When bone marrow is stimulated, with the help of special drugs, a large number of stem cells pours out of the marrow and floods the bloodstream. Stem cells are difficult to distinguish from lymphocytes, and until a few years ago there was no way to find them. Scientists discovered that stem cells had a special molecule on their cell membrane, CD34, which they could use to identify them.

To harvest stem cells, blood is allowed to circulate from the patient through a special machine, where white blood cells and stem cells are separated and removed and then the rest of the blood is returned to the patient. This takes about three hours. Using CD34 as a stem-cell identifier, the total number of harvested stem cells is counted. If the yield is insufficient, the painless procedure is repeated twenty-four hours later. Frozen stem cells are then stored in liquid nitrogen. If required, they are returned to the patient, like the BMT, just as if the patient were receiving a blood transfusion. Unlike lymphoma and leukemia, stem cell transplantation for patients with metastatic breast and other cancers is still experimental.

Alternative Medicine

Cancer patients try alternative medicine less often than patients with other diseases. "Alternative medicine" is a term used in North America to describe unproven remedies and techniques. More than two dozen medical schools and hospitals in North America have developed programs to study it.

Alternative medicine includes "complementary" medicine, in which therapy (such as relaxation) is used in conjunction with, rather than instead of, conventional treatment. Relaxation techniques are prescribed by practitioners and used by thousands of patients, because they produce a sense of well-being. A problem arises when such techniques are used as an alternative to conventional therapy; then they can be dangerous.

Diet, nutrition, hands-on healing methods, folk remedies, and herbal medicine are all used by patients as alternative medicine. Gradually, complementary medicine is partnering mainstream medicine. Some techniques that were at one time regarded as alternative are no longer stigmatized; acupuncture and homeopathy are examples. Others are downright quackery, and often patients cannot tell the difference.

Some cancer patients, especially those who are terminally ill, will grasp at straws and try unproven remedies. They and their families will say that they have nothing to lose (except money). Regrettably, they keep the charlatans and quacks, who give them false hope, in business. There are also misguided patients who seek alternative treatment at a relatively early stage and miss the opportunity for cure by conventional medicine.

During the past century numerous alternative anticancer treatments have come and gone without success. Undoubtedly, the most publicized, useless, and fraudulent drug was Laetrile. For fifty years nonmedical and some medical practitioners touted it as a "natural cure." Its advocates made amazing claims and succeeded in getting it legalized in 1977 in the United States. However, after extensive study and enormous expense, the National Cancer Institute finally put Laetrile, and those with a vested interest in this drug, out of business in the early 1980s. Some new approaches to cancer therapy appear in chapter 14.

Bibliography

Antman, K. When are bone marrow transplants considered? *Scientific American* 275 (1996) 90–91.

Armitage, J.O. Bone marrow transplantation. *New England Journal of Medicine* 330, 12 (1994):827–38.

Aulas, J.J. Alternative cancer treatments. *Scientific American* 275 (1996):126–27.

Buckman, R. *What you really need to know about cancer.* London: Macmillan, 1996.

Cassileth, B.R., and C.C. Chapman. Alternative and complementary cancer therapies. *Cancer* 77 (1996):1026–34.

Dallinger, M., E.H. Rosenbaum, and G. Cable. *Everyone's guide to cancer therapy* 3rd edition. Kansas City: Andrews & McMeel, 1998.

Foley, K.M. Controlling the pain of cancer. *Scientific American* 275 (1996):128–29.

Goldenberg, D.M. *Cancer therapy with radiolabeled antibodies.* Boca Raton, Fla.: CRC Press, 1995.

Greenwald, P. Chemoprevention of cancer. *Scientific American* 275 (1996):64–67.

Hellman, S., and E.E. Vokes. Advancing current treatments for cancer. *Scientific American* 275 (1996):84–89.

Holland, J.C. Cancer's psychological challenges. *Scientific American* 275 (1996):122–25.

Jacox, A., D.B. Carr, and R. Payne. New clinical-practice guidelines for the management of pain in patients with cancer. *New England Journal of Medicine* 330, 9 (1994):651–55.

Janssen, W.F. Cancer quackery—the past in the present. *Seminars in Oncology* 6, 4 (1979): 526–36.

Kaplan, H.S. Historic milestones in radiobiology and radiation therapy. *Seminars in Oncology* 6, 4 (1979):479–89.

Kinzler, K.W., and B. Vogelstein. Cancer therapy meets p53. *New England Journal of Medicine*. 331, 1 (1994):49–50.

Lichter, A.S., and T.S. Lawrence. Recent advances in radiation oncology. *New England Journal of Medicine* 332, 6, (1995):371–9.

Old, L.J. Immunotherapy and cancer. *Scientific American* 275 (1996):102–9.

Oliff, A., J.B. Gibbs, and F. McCormick. New molecular targets for cancer therapy. *Scientific American* 275 (1996):110–15.

Passamani, E. Clinical trials—Are they ethical? *New England Journal of Medicine* 324 (1991):1589–92.

Steller, H. Mechanisms and genes of cellular suicide. *Science* 267, 5203 (1995): 1145–49.

Zubrod, C.G. Historic milestones in curative chemotherapy. *Seminars in Oncology* 6, 4 (1995):490–505.

Internet Sources

Alternative therapies: http://members.aol.com/MIND2BODY/mind2body/html

Clinical trials: http://www.centerwatch.com/BACKGRND.html
http://www.cyber.nl/cancernet/400109.html

CHAPTER 12

Where to Get More Information

When patients learn that they have cancer, they and their relatives are often numbed, confused, angry, and depressed. After the initial panic settles and they start to think objectively, most patients have dozens of questions. As the first queries are answered, more and more questions come to mind. Initially, the source of information is the doctor who breaks the news. The family doctor who sees only a few new cancer patients each year may not have enough information to answer specific detailed questions. The surgeon or cancer specialist or one of the medical team will answer these. Large hospitals and medical centers have oncology units staffed by specialist doctors and nurses, often with links to social workers, psychiatrists, psychologists, dietitians, physiotherapists, and other medical specialists. These experts can provide advice on the special problems of an individual's disease and its treatment.

Many patients want to think as little as possible about their disease. They wish to get on with their lives and leave the medical decisions to the cancer specialists. Some patients wish to participate to varying degrees in the decisions and plans related to their treatment. Often these patients want to delve deeply into their condition, and apart from a natural curiosity about their own particular disease, they become fascinated by the whole topic of cancer. What causes it? How does it grow and spread? What alternative treatments are available? Will their children get it? What is the prognosis? Fortunately, it is now easier than ever to get information about cancer and its treatment. Some patients will not wish to discuss their illness with others, apart from their family and close friends. Others will talk freely and join support groups, caring for patients with cancers similar to their own.

Health sections in large bookstores sometimes have a small selection of books on cancer written for the layperson. These are self-help books and often target patients with specific cancers. Despite the prevalence of cancer and the importance of the topic, it is remarkable how few books explain in lay language what cancer is. Medical libraries have huge sections on the general aspects of cancer, and they usually carry many books on specific cancers and their treatment. They also carry an excellent range of cancer specialist journals. Medical library fare is written in medical and technical jargon and make heavy reading for nonmedics.

Many towns, cities, and communities have self-help groups in which patients and relatives can discuss all aspects of their disease and learn how others cope with the illness and its accompanying social complications (or perceived complications). Invited speakers address them on individual topics. For many patients such groups play an important part in their lives. Friendships are made and troubles are shared. National and international cancer societies supply booklets and often provide a phone-in advice service.

The revolution in computer technology has placed a mountain of information on the Internet, distributed on the World Wide Web (WWW). If you have access to the Internet, this is by far the best and most comprehensive source of cancer information. Furthermore, much of the material is written in nonmedical language. By any imaginable standard, this facility is impressive. The National Cancer Institute (NCI) and many world-renowned cancer centers put information on the Internet, on all aspects of cancer. It is available in separate formats suitable for doctors and patients. Information is updated monthly. Breakthroughs related to cancer, genetics, therapy and the latest information on clinical trials are announced daily. You can browse through advice on social problems, medical insurance, and much more. Professional writers who have had cancer write some of the articles. Internet sites contain information on childhood cancers, and some of the articles have even been written by children. The Internet is growing at a such a rapid rate that even since I began writing this book, many new medical and dozens of cancer information sites were added, often every few months.

Internet users can send questions on any topic under the sun to the Internet community in general and wait for replies. You can, as it were, listen in to conversations as questions and answers go back and forth daily on your computer screen. If you wish to participate in a discussion, you simply type your message on the screen and push a button or click the mouse. Patients send tips on what has helped them in particular situations. If you are shy about having 30 million viewers look at your specific problem, you can send a message by electronic mail (e-mail), privately, to any other person with an e-mail address. It will cost you only a few cents, even if that other person lives at the far end of the planet. Various "news groups" discuss specific cancer topics and issues; others are more general.

Since anybody with a computer and a modem can dial the Internet and deposit information there, the potential for misinformation on the Internet from all sorts of crackpots is great. There is no censorship. Medical information deposited in the Internet by cancer societies, hospitals, medical centers, and governments or their agencies is highly reliable and is written clearly in essays and summaries. Most patients want to read the information in this format.

Patients can also read research information on their particular problem in the Medline database. Medline is compiled by the National Library of Congress in Washington, D.C., and contains an abstract of most major articles published since 1966. It even contains English abstracts of articles published in other languages. This remarkable database provides vital information for health specialists throughout the world and is updated monthly. The world of biomedicine publishes 25,000 journals yearly, and although Medline does not include every journal, it includes every serious journal containing significant clinical information relevant to cancer. Until recently, only academics with university mainframe computers could pull information from Medline. Now anyone with a desktop computer can access the database. It is available in many formats, including CD-ROM, and it is on the Internet. It is now free. Some computer experience is necessary to know how to interrogate the database intelligently.

For most patients Medline is not very useful, since its information is too technical. Sometimes bewildered patients or relatives arrive in the doctor's office with miles of computer printout, containing the results of cancer studies from Boston, London, or Tokyo. In general, Medline searches carried out indiscriminately on particular diseases or treatments are not useful, as they rarely address the combination of variables or circumstances pertinent to an individual patient. Far more useful is the summarized information provided by the cancer societies and medical centers. They give invaluable advice on all aspects of cancer management, and patients can print out their Internet pages for future reference. If they prefer, they can quickly save the information in their computers for later use.

Internet sites also provide hypertext links to other information centers. A hypertext link is simply a color-coded word or phrase. The user points the cursor (arrowhead) at the link word and presses the mouse button. Within a few seconds he or she can browse a new Internet site. Because most Internet information is provided by American universities and institutions, it is biased, understandably, toward Americans. Most contacts and information centers are located in the United States. Nevertheless, cancer information, dealing with general or specific medical problems, is relevant to patients everywhere in the world.

Bookstores and librarians have their own publishing databases, and they can find information easily and quickly. They will help you find a suitable book. If the book you require is not in stock, most bookstores will gladly order it for you.

The National Cancer Institute in Washington, D.C. runs the Cancer Information Service (CIS), which provides a nationwide telephone service for cancer patients, the public, and health-care professionals. They answer questions in English and Spanish and will send written information on request. Their toll-free number is 1-800-4-cancer (1-800-422-6237). A list of important World Wide Web addresses is in the appendix. Useful support agencies are also in the appendix.

I would strongly advise anyone who requires detailed information on any aspect of cancer to go on the Internet. Those who do not know how to use the Internet, or who do not have access to this wonder of the decade, will be thrilled and delighted at the experience. The small effort required to learn how to use the Internet will be rewarded. Although the Internet has 30 million viewers worldwide and 30 percent of American homes now have computers, most cancer patients still do not have a connection to the Internet. For most patients, the Internet and the World Wide Web are just names they read or hear about occasionally. These patients should get useful advice and help from their friendly librarian. Undoubtedly, libraries will all eventually provide Internet facilities for the public. Already some libraries do so. (See appendix.)

Bibliography

Annas, G.J. Informed consent, cancer, and truth in prognosis. *New England Journal of Medicine* 330, 3 (1994):223–25. [Published erratum appears in 330, 9 (1994): 651.]

Baldwin, F., and S. McInerney. *Infomedicine: A consumer's guided to the latest medical research.* Boston: Little, Brown, 1996.

Buckman, R. *What you really need to know about cancer.* London: Macmillan, 1996.

Christakis, N.A., J.J. Escarce. Survival of Medicare patients after enrollment in hospice programs. *New England Journal of Medicine.* 335, 3 (1996):172–78.

Dallinger, M., E.H. Rosenbaum, and G. Cable. *Everyone's guide to cancer therapy.* Kansas City: Andrews & McMeel, 1998.

Internet Sources

http://www.elibrary.com/
http://oncolink.upenn.edu/
http://www.cancer.org/
http://infoventures.com/cancer/
http://oncolink.upenn.edu/resources/association/org.html

CHAPTER 13

Cancer Screening

The overall goal of screening is to reduce mortality in populations at risk for cancer. This is accomplished by detecting dysplastic changes before they become malignant, or by detecting very early invasive cancers that have an excellent prognosis. Screening programs target asymptomatic individuals. The ultimate purpose of screening programs is to give the public the opportunity to avoid death from cancer. In practice, how realistic is this goal? For some cancers, screening succeeds very well; for others there is great debate and controversy over the efficacy of screening. Screening for some cancers is a waste of time and money. Acute leukemia, for example, has an acute onset, is widespread at the time of diagnosis, and often has no recognizable premalignant phase. There are no useful screening programs for such malignancies. When reading about screening for cancer, try to identify whether the author is writing about screening an individual patient for cancer or screening an entire population. The distinction is important.

Patients and doctors regard cancer screening as a benefit to the individual. However, the screening program organizers and sponsors (usually government agencies) have quite a different idea about its purpose. They regard it as a benefit to large populations: it is a public health issue, and it concerns society in general. Cancer (population) screening is enormously expensive. Doctors, nurses, epidemiologists, paramedical staff, administrators, computer workers, and clerical workers generate volumes of data. The specific purpose is to reduce overall mortality for the screened population. The idea of benefit to the individual is often lost in the general strategy of public health decisions. Apart from reduced mortality, other benefits include the lesser cost of treating patients with early rather than advanced cancer and reduced morbidity e.g. breast "lumpectomy" rather than mastectomy.

Patients with smaller cancers need less surgery, less hospital time, and fewer investigations. Societies would be healthier if cancers were detected while they were small and still localized. Governments studying cost-benefit ratios need to control how much tax money they spend. They have an obligation to ensure that their health-care budget is put to the best use. Public issues like immunization, good sanitation, good nutrition, and control of infectious diseases have (deservedly) a higher priority than cancer screening in all countries. However, after basic public health programs are stable, then prevention of specific cancers is a worthwhile pursuit.

Screening a patient in the doctor's office changes the rationale and sometimes diagnostic reasoning may be slightly blurred. "What is good for the country is not necessarily what is good for my patient"—the doctor reasons. What the doctor needs now for this special person is a test as sensitive and specific as possible. If necessary, the doctor will order a battery of tests. Population economics are less important. The concern for the individual overrides all else.

Nevertheless, in general, those tests that have proven their value in large population screening studies tend to be the best tests also for the individual, and those tests that are of no value in screening tend not to be helpful for the individual. The main controversies between population and individual screening tend to involve borderline areas such as mammography for women under the age of 50 and prostate specific antigen as a test for prostate cancer. While these tests have not proven themselves in population screening, their use for individual patients is well accepted. There is often one major difference between population screening and screening the individual. The person in the doctor's office is probably there because of some symptom, whereas population screening concentrates on asymptomatic people. When the criteria for screening are changed from asymptomatic to symptomatic people, the statistical probability of finding an abnormal test also changes.

Which are the most successful cancer screening programs, and what are the obstacles and difficulties to screening? The criteria for a successful screening program are: (1) the disease should be relatively common, i.e., have a high prevalence in the community, (2) there should be a good treatment for the condition, (3) the screening test used should be inexpensive, and (4) the test should be highly sensitive and highly specific. If I have a screening test performed and I am told that it is negative, I may go away happy in the belief that I do not have cancer. I may not have heard of false negative results and may not realize that a negative result is no guarantee that I do not have cancer. What a negative result really means is that there is a strong statistical probability that I do not have cancer. Likewise, if I have a positive result, I may not understand that all screening tests have some false positives, and that this test will need some form of confirmatory test before cancer is diagnosed.

A test with perfect sensitivity would detect everyone who had the disease, i.e., it would miss nobody. No person with disease would slip through this screening net. A test with perfect specificity would ensure that all individuals with a positive test would have the disease. Such a test would not be confused or confounded by other factors—it would not give a false positive result. A test with perfect sensitivity and perfect specificity does not exist for any disease. Doctors choose screening tests that have a high degree of sensitivity. This inevitably means that they sometimes get false positive results. A positive screening test must be followed up by a confirmatory diagnostic test.

Malignant melanoma, to explore one example, has a high prevalence in Australia, among the fair-skinned Celtic population in particular. Screening for melanoma is fairly simple and inexpensive. Citizens are taught the danger signals for suspicious skin lesions. They are taught how to examine themselves, with the use of mirrors to visualize difficult areas of the body, and to report to their doctors if they detect some suspicious abnormality. Obviously, many patients will report abnormalities that are not malignant. These are the false positive cases. The doctor will examine the patient, eliminate the innocuous mimics, detect the true positive cases, and confirm these by pathologic examination. Although false positives in a program like this are common, no harm is done. Such a program is simple, inexpensive, and without significant adverse implications for the health services.

How effective screening is depends on what percentage of the population will examine itself. Most screening programs require the participation of about 70 percent to be effective. If only a small percentage of the target group follows the screening advice, then the total number of prevented cancers will have very little effect on the overall mortality rate. So, although screening will benefit greatly those screened and save their lives, the official screening program will be deemed an overall failure as a public health project. For skin cancer screening, the only major financial outlay is for the advertising campaign.

Unlike skin cancer, screening for breast cancer is very expensive, and a high rate of patient compliance is essential for a successful program. Many worldwide studies have evaluated the effect of screening on mortality, sometimes with very different results. Some of the conflicting results have come from studies that have taken place decades apart. The later studies, e.g., in mammographic breast screening programs, used far more advanced and sophisticated equipment. Often these studies are not exactly comparable because they use different methodologies. Despite these differences, there is an emerging consensus that screening is useful for specific cancers in specific situations, such as breast screening in defined age groups.

The original idea of cancer screening focused on screening large asymptomatic populations at risk for a particular cancer. This is still what most people mean when they talk about screening for cancer. More recently, however, the concept of screening has been extended to include individuals and families at risk for specific cancers. Sometimes this process takes the form of long-term surveillance. A few benign diseases have a propensity to evolve into cancer, usually after many years. Polyps are benign tumors that may become malignant if they are not removed. Even when they are removed, they sometimes recur. Many patients with polyps require long-term surveillance. Most polyps occur sporadically and should not be confused with the genetic disease, familial polyposis coli. This condition inevitably progresses to cancer unless the colon and its polyps are removed. Patients cured of colonic cancer are at increased risk for developing more colonic cancers at a later date, and so they also are put on a surveillance program.

Barrett's esophagus and ulcerative colitis are inflammatory conditions with an increased risk. The screening procedure for these intestinal conditions is endoscopy and biopsy. The endoscopist, usually a gastroenterologist or surgeon, passes an optical tube-like instrument into the lumen of the intestine, where he or she can visualize directly the surface of the intestine. This allows the endoscopist to direct the biopsy forceps at any visible abnormality.

In recent years the possibility of screening for genetic cancers has appeared on the horizon. The revolution in molecular biology has brought new information on the genetic predisposition to a variety of cancers. Now DNA tests are developing rapidly to identify asymptomatic individuals and families at risk. A few cancers in particular have been studied in detail. These include familial breast cancer and hereditary nonpolyposis colon cancer.

Hereditary genetic mutations cause approximately 10 percent of breast cancers. Two genes called BRCA1 and BRCA2 are responsible for most of them. Even women without a family history may harbor these mutations. A woman with a family history and one of these mutations has an 80 percent lifetime risk of developing breast cancer. Naturally, many women with a family history will be concerned about their risk and may want to avail themselves of genetic screening tests. Although DNA screening tests are widely available for nonmalignant diseases, such as cystic fibrosis, genetic tests for breast cancer are not quite ready yet for widespread consumer use.

In the rest of this chapter screening programs for various cancers are discussed.

Colon Cancer

The large intestine comprises the colon and its distal segment, the rectum. As mentioned in chapter 6, in the United States each year almost

140,000 new cases of colorectal cancer are diagnosed, and it kills 55,000, making it the second leading cause (after lung cancer) of cancer mortality. The incidence is slightly higher in men, and most cases are diagnosed after the age of 50. If it is diagnosed at an early, localized stage, the five-year survival rate is nearly 100 percent. For patients presenting with advanced stage disease (spread to liver) there is virtually no chance of cure. Those patients with intermediate-stage disease have a five-year survival rate of approximately 60 percent–80 percent. Almost all patients who survive for five years, without evidence of recurrent disease, are cured.

For decades, we have known that most colon cancers arise from small benign tumors, called polyps. Only a tiny percentage of polyps eventually turn malignant, and the main purpose of screening for colon cancer is to detect and remove these precancerous growths. Even if they have become malignant, patients benefit greatly by early removal of localized cancers. Theoretically, screening for polyps and early cancer should reduce mortality.

There are two major screening tests for colorectal cancer. One is easy to perform and it is cheap and highly acceptable to patients; the other is difficult, expensive, and not pleasant. Cancers and polyps have a tendency to leak tiny amounts of blood from their surface. This blood mixes with feces and can be detected by a very simple test called a fecal occult (meaning hidden) blood test. The test is easy to perform and cheap, and it has a high acceptability rate. The patient just smears a small amount of feces on a preconditioned card and mails it to a pathology laboratory. Unfortunately, it is too sensitive and gives too many false positive results. The overall evidence is that an annual fecal occult blood test can reduce mortality from colorectal cancer. However, the high incidence of false positive tests severely limits its usefulness.

The second test is sigmoidoscopy. A sigmoidoscope is an optical tube-like instrument that is inserted through the anus, into the rectum and left side of the colon. Here the entire surface of the rectum and left side of the colon can be examined visually. Small polyps are snipped away and cancers are biopsied. The rationale for confining the procedure to the left side of the colon is based on the fact that most polyps and cancers occur here; as a screening procedure, this is quite effective. It is possible also to use a longer instrument, a colonoscope, to visualize the entire colon.

Virtually all screening studies using sigmoidoscopy prove that this is an effective method for reducing colorectal mortality. As you can imagine, the procedure is not embraced with rapture and enthusiasm by the public. Patient acceptability is crucial to any successful screening program. Nevertheless, it is acceptable to some individuals and while sigmoidoscopy may never catch on as a general population screening procedure it will undoubtedly benefit those prepared to undergo such an examination. Individuals with a family history of colon cancer or patients with a past history of colonic polyps benefit most from sigmoidoscopy. Future studies propose to evaluate the usefulness of detecting DNA mutations in feces as a screening technique.

Breast Cancer

Breast cancer in males is rare. It makes up less than 1 percent of all breast cancers. Therefore, all discussion on the topic of breast cancer screening is confined to females. Three techniques are used to screen for breast cancer: (1) breast examination by a physician or nurse, (2) self-examination, and (3) mammography. Breast cancer must reach a critical size, usually about 1cm, before the patient or doctor can feel it. Other factors, such as the size of the breast and the proximity of the tumor to the surface, also determine how easy or difficult it is to palpate (feel) a tumor. Obviously, superficial tumors are easier to find than deeply situated tumors, and they are easier to identify in small breasts. Most palpable cancers are invasive tumors, i.e., they have progressed beyond the in situ stage. In contrast, mammography can detect preinvasive carcinoma in situ and invasive cancers too small to feel.

We have strong evidence that screening by mammography reduces overall mortality from breast cancer in the age group 50 to 69. However, there is still controversy and debate over its value in the age group 40 to 49; there is insufficient evidence to show that it reduces population mortality in this age group. Over the age of 70 we do not have enough information to decide one way or the other.

Despite the seemingly obvious conclusion that examination of the breast for small cancers by doctors or patients should reduce mortality, such is not the case. There is no evidence that such examinations by patient or doctor reduces mortality in a screened population. Of course, individuals may and do benefit from finding small early cancers. Its lack of usefulness refers to the overall statistics for the screened population.

The incidence of breast cancer has been increasing gradually over the past fifty years. Up to 1987 it was the prime cancer killer in women. Now it takes second place to lung cancer. In the United States, 185,000 new cases are diagnosed each year and 46,000 women die from this scourge. Early diagnosis accounts for most of the increase. Breast cancer has a high public profile and more and more women are conscious of the benefit of early diagnosis. Cancer societies and health departments worldwide have strong cancer-awareness campaigns and health-education programs, advocating the use of mammography for the prevention of breast-cancer deaths.

The incidence of breast cancer is lower in United States blacks than in whites. However, blacks have a higher mortality rate. When you look at the reasons for this, one stands out immediately. At the time of diagnosis, blacks have a more advanced stage of disease. So their survival rates, from the time of diagnosis to death, is short. Whites have a better chance of cure, not because they are genetically privileged, but because they are diagnosed at an earlier, more curable stage.

Breast screening has had a checkered career, with many hotly debated arguments for and against. Gradually the advocates are winning, and many cancer societies throughout the western world support mammographic screening. A number of countries, including the United Kingdom, Sweden, and the Netherlands, now fund national breast-screening programs. Other countries are following and are in the process of setting up the huge infrastructures necessary to fund national programs.

At one stage, some scientists feared that certain patients were highly susceptible to radiation damage, and that even tiny amounts of mammography radiation might be sufficient to cause breast cancer. There was a scare that mammography might be doing more harm than good. Many studies show that such fears are unfounded. Mammography is safe.

Mammography is a specialized X-ray procedure. Its great value is in identifying in situ (preinvasive) cancers and cancers too small to feel. With in situ cancers there is a deposit of calcium within the ducts containing the cancer cells. Calcium has a tendency to deposit in tumor cells and stands out from surrounding soft tissues. Just as calcium makes bones easy to see on X-rays, so too fine, subtle calcium deposits enable the trained radiologist to pick out very early malignant change. Because a number of benign conditions can mimic the mammographic appearance of malignancy, a confirmatory diagnostic test is necessary before treatment—either a fine needle aspirate or a small biopsy.

Not all in situ cancers calcify, and these can be missed in the mammogram. These are the false negatives. In all screening programs there is a follow-up recall examination after two or three years. A slowly growing tumor, one that was invisible originally, may have the tell-tale signs of malignancy two years later.

Some cancers never calcify. The radiologist may still be able to identify them by their irregular density and growth pattern on the mammogram. The ability to discriminate these small cancers from normal breast tissues is often very difficult and depends on the relative density of the normal surrounding breast tissue. If the surrounding breast contains an abundance of fibrous tissue and glands, as is normal in younger patients, it may be impossible to see the difference in radiological contrast between tumor and normal tissue. This is one reason why mammography is less useful in younger women. Older patients (over 50) tend to have more fat and less fibrous and glandular breast tissue. In these breasts, tumors are more easily identified.

Sometimes, clinically obvious, palpable tumors cannot be seen on X-rays because of the lack of contrast between tumor and normal tissue. Luckily this situation is uncommon, and it does not interfere with the overall effectiveness of breast-screening programs.

Huge technical improvements in mammographic technique, better study design, improved overall quality control, and better training for radiologists contribute greatly to the success of more recent screening programs.

Regarding patient acceptability, mammography has some problems. Many women complain of varying degrees of discomfort. To get good quality X-ray images (essential for interpretation) it is necessary to compress the breasts. A pair of mammographic plates squeezes each breast between them until the breast has an almost flat contour. Understandably, patients would prefer a more comfortable procedure; radiologists and manufacturers are trying to design more comfortable machines.

Researchers believe that many of the problems with interpretation of mammograms can be overcome by newer magnetic resonance imaging (MRI) techniques. At present MRI is impractical for screening procedures. Too few scanners are available and the procedure is too time-consuming and too expensive for nondiagnostic (i.e., screening) use. However, when we look at the rapidly advancing knowledge and applications in computer technology, it would be foolish to dismiss the possible contributions of MRI to screening in the future.

Cancer of the Cervix

Cervical cancer provides the classical model for cancer prevention. Premalignant cellular changes precede the onset of in situ and invasive cancer, usually by many years. Because the cervix is an external surface (relatively speaking), doctors or nurses can examine it and remove cells directly from its surface. Specially trained cytotechnologists screen these cells microscopically to identify very early abnormalities. This is the Papanicolaou (Pap) smear test. Malignant or premalignant changes are confirmed by biopsy. In the United States, 16,000 patients with invasive cervical cancer are diagnosed each year and almost 5,000 die from the disease. In theory, it should be possible to prevent these deaths.

Since the early 1950s the incidence and mortality rates for invasive cervical cancer have fallen by about 70 percent in the western world. Much of the credit for this goes to cervical screening, and many screening program successes are due to widespread acceptance by the public. Success is correlated with the intensity of screening efforts, and those communities with the greatest participation have the greatest reduction in mortality rates. Statistics for cervical cancer in the developing world are wildly different from those of western societies. Worldwide almost 500,000 new cases of cervical cancer are recorded annually; approximately 80 percent of these are in developing countries. In many countries it is the most common female lethal cancer. Despite its long history and proven track record, cervical screening still has many deficiencies as a screening system.

Interpretation of subtle premalignant changes is difficult and requires an expertly trained cytotechnologist. Cytology is labor-intensive. Each smear must be examined slowly and carefully. Each abnormality must be double-checked with another expert, usually a pathologist. Because it is labor-intensive, human fatigue must be minimized by restricting the number of cases any cytotechnologist can screen per unit of time. Normally this is about eighty slides per day. Otherwise, small but possibly significant abnormalities will be missed. Furthermore, to reduce the possibility of missing such abnormalities, about 10 percent of the negative cases will be screened again. A variety of such quality-assurance procedures bolsters a high quality of performance in laboratories throughout the western world.

Despite the best efforts and conscientiousness of all concerned, a small percentage of false negatives occur, even in the most competent laboratories. Making sure that the laboratory performs optimally is only part of the screening process. The screening organization and management must run smoothly. Patients need reminders, and more reminders, to continue in a follow-up program. Sometimes reminders are not enough. If someone does not respond to a recall it may be important to find out why. Has she moved to another location or changed her name or possibly died? Each step of the screening process must be continually reviewed and monitored. Each step has its own quality-assurance techniques. Each step must be integrated into the overall structure and organization of the screening program.

Participants in the ideal cervical screening program should have their first screening in early adulthood or late teens, and this should be repeated at every two, three, or five years. The protection offered by screening decreases as the duration between tests gets longer, or as the frequency of testing decreases. Although the degree of protection is proportional to the number of screenings, the marginal effectiveness decreases with an increasing number of screenings; so does the cost-effectiveness of the test. The incidence of cervical cancer in women screened at one- or two-year intervals is reduced by more than 90 percent; at five-year intervals it is approximately 80 percent; and at ten-year intervals it is approximately 65 percent.

Even in 40- to 50-year-old women there is a reduced incidence of 25 percent associated with screening just once.

The time-honored test for cervical screening is the Pap smear. Dr. George Papanicolaou introduced the test more than fifty years ago. Because it is labor-intensive, slow, expensive, and subjective, doctors, scientists, and administrators are continually searching for a better screening method. Two new techniques, one computer-based, the other biotechnology-based, currently show great promise.

The first technique captures a large number of microscopic images on computer, and using a neural network (a computerized type of artificial intelligence) compares the screened cells with known normal and abnormal cells. Furthermore, it displays detected abnormalities as multiple simultaneous high-resolution images. A cytotechnologist or pathologist reviews these images quickly on the computer screens, and if necessary reviews the original microscopic slide. This system has proven its ability to detect abnormalities in a research setting. However, its real value may be in the rescreening, quality-assurance step.

The second technique is based on the fact that a very large proportion of cervical cancers and precancers contain oncogenic subtypes of the human papilloma virus (HPV). DNA specific for these subtypes can be identified by a powerful molecular biology technique, called the polymerase chain reaction (PCR). PCR technology is now standard in most biology laboratories throughout the world. Although conceptually this molecular biology technique is sophisticated and high-tech, in practice it can be automated and carried out by relatively unskilled personnel, and multiple samples can be screened rapidly. Investigators and health agencies are evaluating the newer techniques and seriously considering them as primary screening procedures. However, for the present, and the foreseeable future, the fifty-year-old Pap test remains the standard.

Prostate Cancer

In contrast to breast cancer, we see and hear little about prostate cancer. Nevertheless, prostate cancer is more common than breast cancer and kills as many patients. In 1996 there were more than 317,000 new cases in the United States and 41,000 deaths. It accounts for 36 percent of all male cancers and 13 percent of male cancer deaths.

There are some striking differences between breast and prostate cancer. The most obvious is the age of the patients. Prostate cancer is uncommon before the age of 50; a considerable percentage of breast cancers devastate women's lives before 50. The incidence and prevalence rates for prostate cancer include a large number of slow-growing nonlethal cancers that require no treatment that often are found incidentally at autopsy. Nevertheless, prostate cancer affects many men between the ages of 50 and 65. The cost to the United States economy annually is $3.7 billion. Of this, $1.3 billion represents indirect costs such as loss of productivity and wages.

As in other screening programs, the goal with prostate screening is to diagnose and treat small, early-stage tumors. The most common, least expensive test for prostate cancer is digital rectal examination by a physician. The physician inserts a finger into the rectum and palpates the prostate gland, through the thin wall of the rectum (the prostate lies just in front of the rectum). Cancer is usually firmer than surrounding normal prostate tissue and it reveals itself to the palpating finger as a firm or hard nodule. Such an abnormality is followed up by a visit to a surgeon or urologist, who performs a needle core biopsy. Ultrasound scanning of the prostate may be helpful in localizing a small nodule.

A new biochemical assay has now become the standard screening technique for prostate cancer. It is the prostate specific antigen (PSA) assay. This has the great advantage that it is noninvasive. All that is required is a simple blood test. Normal prostate cells secrete PSA in very low quantities, and this spills over into the bloodstream, where it can be measured. Cancers produce greater amounts of PSA, which are reflected by higher levels in the blood. The amount of PSA in the blood usually correlates with the amount of tumor present. Small elevations usually indicate a small, localized (curable) tumor and large elevations often indicate that the patient has metastases.

In theory, PSA is in many ways an ideal screening tool. It has a high degree of sensitivity and specificity, and it is reliable. It is an excellent method for screening individual patients. However, when applied to populations, it has not passed the ultimate test; PSA screening has not proven that it can reduce overall mortality from prostate cancer. Nevertheless, the American Cancer Society and the American Urological Association recommend screening for prostate cancer in men over 50 years old who have a life expectancy of at least ten years. Those with a family history should start at age 40.

Lung Cancer

Smoking causes approximately 90 percent of lung cancers. Smoking also contributes significantly to cancer of the mouth, throat, and larynx (voice box). It is ironic that screening procedures are not very helpful in identifying lung cancer, but these cancers are preventable by avoiding cigarettes. Researchers believe that smoking also contributes to cancer of the esophagus, bladder, cervix, kidney, and pancreas. The dangers from smoke inhalation are not confined to smokers. Some of the friends, family, and coworkers who are exposed to long-term "passive" smoking may also be at risk for lung cancer. Epidemiologists estimate that exposure to environmental tobacco smoke, i.e., passive smoking, accounts for many thousand lung cancers in nonsmokers each year. This is a highly controversial topic with major implications for employers, owners of shopping malls, and those with responsibility for the health and safety of all occupants in buildings. However, recent evidence suggests that early statistics on victims of passive smoking are possibly exaggerated.

The theory behind screening for lung cancer is similar to that for other cancers. Find the precancerous growth, or a very early tumor before it has spread, and you should be able to cure the patient. Two methods have been tried, chest X-rays and cytological examination of sputum for dysplastic or malignant cells. Neither procedure is useful. Population screening for lung cancer is deemed largely futile and has been all but abandoned. Most experts agree that putting the money into health education, to prevent young people from taking up the habit, is money better spent. Screening enthusiasts may soon study DNA mutations in sputum to see whether these could provide a useful screening technique for lung cancer.

Cancer of the Ovary

Like the lungs and prostate, the ovaries are hidden in a body cavity. The prognosis for small, early ovarian cancers is excellent, with a five-year survival of approximately 90 percent. However, fewer than 25 percent of ovarian cancers are diagnosed while they are localized. The overall five-year survival is less than 40 percent. Each year 26,600 new cases are diagnosed and 14,000 patients die.

Screening methods for early cancer include physical (pelvic) examination, ultrasound examination of the ovaries, and measurement of a cancer marker in the blood, called CA-125. None of these tests is of proven value as a population screening method. CA-125 is valuable as a marker of recurrent disease and is used routinely to monitor a patient's progress after treatment.

Cancer of the Testis

The success of testicular cancer therapy is one of the most spectacular achievements in the modern oncology era. Most patients are cured, even those with metastases at the time of diagnosis. As usual, however, the more extensive the disease, the more difficult it is to achieve a cure.

Self-examination, detection by physical examination, and possibly ultrasound offer potential screening methods. At present there is no evidence that population screening can reduce mortality. However, special risk groups such as young men with cryptorchidism (failure of the testis to descend from the abdomen into the scrotum, during embryogenesis) or Klinefelter's syndrome (a chromosomal abnormality associated with maldevelopment of the testes) should benefit from early screening and diagnosis. This cancer illustrates one of the basic difficulties with the philosophy of screening. Testicular cancer is rare; it accounts for only 1 percent of all male cancers. The mathematics and statistics of population screening indicate that screening for rare diseases is unlikely to reduce population mortality, particularly when treatment is so effective.

Cancer of the Stomach

The incidence of gastric cancer has decreased dramatically in the western world since 1930. However, Japan and other Asian countries have a much higher incidence. The reduced incidence in the western world is attributed to changes in our diet and particularly in the way food is preserved. In Japan, screening has significantly reduced the incidence of gastric cancer. There is insufficient evidence to show that screening is effective in western countries.

Skin Cancer

The commonest skin cancers are basal cell and squamous cell carcinomas. However, these are slow-growing, indolent tumors that are readily treated by surgery. They rarely kill patients, and so there is little rationale for population screening—at least not as a preventive strategy to reduce cancer deaths. Less common but lethal is the malignant melanoma. The patient can recognize malignant melanoma by looking at his or her skin. In its early stage it is completely curable. Fair-skinned individuals, particularly those exposed to sunlight for prolonged periods, are especially at risk. Because Australia has a high proportion of fair-skinned Celts, it has a large population of susceptible individuals. Screening for melanoma in Australia and in Scotland has successfully reduced mortality from melanoma. In Australia sixty years of rising mortality from melanoma has stabilized, and it has started to fall among women. Success is due to education and screening and to the preventive "slip, slop, slap" technique—slip on a shirt, slop on a sunscreen, and slap on a hat.

Bibliography

Austoker, J. Melanoma: Prevention and early diagnosis. *British Medical Journal* 308, 6945 (1994): 1682–86.

Flehinger, B.J., M. Kimmel, T. Polyak, and M.R. Melamed. Screening for lung cancer. The Mayo Lung Project revisited. *Cancer* 72, 5 (1993):1573–80.

Jonsen, A.R., S.J. Durfy, W. Burke, and A.G. Motulsky. The advent of the "unpatients." *Nature Medicine* 2, 6 (1996):622–24.

La Vecchia, C., F. Levi, S. Franceschi. Screening for cancer, 1995: An update. *Annals in Oncology* 6, 6 (1995):537–541.

Liu, E.T. From the molecule to public health. *New England Journal of Medicine* 329, 27 (1993):2028–29.

Maranto, G. Should women in their 40s have mammograms? *Scientific American* 275 (1996):79.

Richart, R.M. Screening. The next century. *Cancer* 76, 10 (1995 suppl.):1919–27.

Sidransky, D. Advances in cancer detection. *Scientific American* 275 (1996):70–75.

Stix, G. Is genetic testing premature? *Scientific American* 275 (1996):107.

Wright, P.A., and D. Wynford-Thomas. Mutations in familial cancer. *Journal of Pathology* 172 (1994):167–70.

Internet Source

http://oncolink.upenn.edu/causeprevent/screening/

CHAPTER 14

The Future

The purpose of research is to answer questions. At first glance, we appear to have only three major questions—what causes cancer, how do we cure it, and how do we prevent it? It is, however, naive and simplistic to think that we can tackle these major questions without asking a thousand smaller questions. Researchers are confident that the answers to the small questions will eventually answer the big questions.

We often equate cancer research with basic fundamental biological research, the type carried out by molecular biologists and biochemists. In practice, the scope of cancer research is much broader. Researchers probe and query every aspect of biology that touches on cancer. They also ask questions about the day-to-day practical problems that invade the life of the cancer patient. Every group of individuals caring for these patients has specific questions. Oncologists want to know the best treatments. Radiologists want to know the best imaging techniques. Pathologists want to know the best diagnostic and prognostic markers. Nurses want to know the best way to care for the patient. Psychiatrists and psychologists want to help patients and their families cope with the additional stresses that come when someone falls victim to cancer. Pharmacologists and chemists want to invent better drugs.

Governments and health agencies around the world carry out many unspectacular but nevertheless very important research programs. Government's role is to identify the best and most cost effective methods for delivering cancer health care to communities. This requires extensive collaboration with public-health authorities, epidemiologists, statisticians, and economists.

The headline-grabbing basic science cancer research, reported in our daily newspapers and on television, is exciting. Research is expensive. The money comes from various sources—governments, cancer societies, universities, and philanthropists all donate. Most western governments allocate part of their budget to health research. Cancer research has a high priority and, like heart disease and AIDS research, gets a moderate slice of the pie.

The United States government spent $2 billion on cancer research in 1996. Still it is not enough.

The politics in government funding of research are complex. Resources are scarce and competition for funds is fierce. Many laboratories and research workers are dedicated to cancer research and their very existence depends on income from research grants. However, researchers working on Alzheimer's disease, AIDS, or schizophrenia feel that their efforts are every bit as worthy as those working with cancer. So, for that matter, do researchers in every other health area.

At the beginning of this chapter I mentioned that two of the main research questions were what was the cause and what was the cure. Amazing progress has been made in the treatment of some cancers, such as testicular cancer, Hodgkin's disease, and the childhood leukemias. Therapy for the common adult cancers on the other hand, such as those involving lung, breast, prostate, colon cancer, and most others, has been disappointing. In chapter 6 we saw that cancer is not one but many diseases. Research into the cause of cancer has been dismal. Most investigations in this area are epidemiological and concentrate on finding links or associations between specific cancers and the environment. With the few notable exceptions mentioned in chapter 6, researchers have made little progress.

In contrast, scientists have made amazing progress in our understanding of the fundamental biology of the cancer cell. At present, this information is mainly of theoretical interest. In the long term, doctors and other health-care workers will translate much of this research into useful therapeutic information. Not only does the world of science believe this, the world of commerce is also convinced. Already stock markets around the world are trading in the new biotechnology industries. Many entrepreneurs, small start-up companies, and pharmaceutical giants think that they are going to get rich or richer on cancer therapy.

The major thrust at present is directed at a deeper understanding of the genetic mechanisms that control cancer growth, invasion, and metastases—and from the therapeutic viewpoint how to neutralize, destroy or alter these genes. Many researchers see the cell cycle and its controlling genes as the key to cancer therapy. Weekly, new research gives us a deeper understanding of the genetic switches that control every step of the cycle. Since the cell cycle is the most important process controlling cell proliferation, it is intuitively satisfying to believe that intense research activity should focus on every ministep of every phase of the cycle. What signals tell a resting cell to start moving? How are these signals processed? What genes need to be activated or inactivated?

New therapeutic tactics aim at specific controls in the cell cycle. Some of the new strategies are novel drug-delivery systems, replacement of defective genes with normal genes, inhibiting messages brought by mRNA from defective genes, and slowing or abolishing tumor angiogenesis. (See chapter 5.)

Anticancer drugs are remarkably efficient at destroying cancer cells. Unfortunately, they are also highly toxic to normal cells. The pharmaceutical industry pours billions of dollars into its effort to produce better drug-delivery systems. Their goal is to produce "magic bullets" that will target and destroy tumor cells but leave normal cells undamaged. Over the years, they have invented various strategies, like tagging drugs or isotopes to antibodies directed against tumor cells, or drugs that block mRNA cell growth signals. These attempts had some experimental success. However, they have not yet made their way into clinical practice.

Chemoprevention is another approach to fighting cancer. Some scientists believe that it may be possible to halt or reverse the process of malignant transformation in individual cells. These studies are still at an experimental stage. They focus on high-risk groups such as those with premalignant conditions, a strong family history of cancer, or risky life-style factors (such as smoking). The results of many ongoing trials are not available yet. All health agencies advocate a well-balanced, low-fat diet, with generous amounts of whole-grain foods, fruit, and vegetables.

Other anticancer strategies include (1) vaccines that stimulate the normal immune system to destroy tumors, (2) drugs that block growth factors or stop them from binding to receptors on the cell surfaces, (3) drugs that inhibit telomerase activity. Scientists at cancer research laboratories around the world are examining genetic-manipulation techniques to induce tumor cells to mature and change back to normal cells. To reverse this process of aberrant evolution is a monumental task.

Each year government research agencies and multinational pharmaceutical and biotechnology companies spend billions of dollars on making tiny breakthroughs in our understanding of cancer. Most researchers are optimistic that step by step cancer will eventually be conquered. Predicting how long it might take is to a large extent guesswork; we can expect it to take many decades at least. Our understanding of the cancer process has grown logarithmically with the recent advances in molecular biology and its applications. The greatest optimists hope that after many baby steps one or two new major discoveries will lead to a new massive leap forward. One day, we may be able to treat cancer as readily as tuberculosis, but first we need to understand it better and in particular to understand what causes it. At one time, the causes of tuberculosis and many other infective diseases were unknown. These were progressive killers, just as cancer is now.

Vaccines may have a role to play in the prevention and treatment of some cancers. As mentioned in chapter 6, certain subtypes of the human papilloma virus (HPV) are strongly linked to cancer of the cervix. Vaccines against these subtypes might prevent these viruses from causing cellular chaos. Already a small preliminary study gave promising results, and a new larger trial has begun. Cancers that are caused by viruses, or those in whose development viruses play a major role, should be preventable and treatable by vaccines. The next few years will tell us whether this is a realistic dream.

Early vaccination successes for malignant melanoma have not been repeated. Nevertheless, in many centers of excellence throughout the world, immunologists continue to devise new anticancer vaccination techniques. The basic idea behind cancer vaccines is to try to get the body's immune system to see the cancer cells as foreign tissue and to destroy them, as it would with transplanted tissue from another person.

Radiotherapists also are major research participants in the war on cancer. They are devising new, safer methods for delivering lethal X-rays to tumors. Some chemicals make tumors more sensitive to X-rays, and radiotherapists are continually trying to find ways to exploit these radiosensitizers.

While most scientific research is aimed at understanding how cancer grows and metastasizes, an entirely different field of research is dedicated to new diagnostic methods. This field of research looks at methods of early diagnosis, the reasoning being that the earlier the diagnosis, the better the chance of cure.

We now have the promise of a novel gene therapy approach not only for cancer but for many inherited diseases. The concept of gene therapy, wherein defective genes are replaced with their normal counterparts, has captured the imagination of scientists and the public. What is gene therapy? Is it useful? Is it available now? The answer to the last question is not at the time of this writing—the end of 1999.

The central idea behind gene therapy is very simple. Insert a fresh normal gene into a cell where one is missing, or replace a defective gene with a perfect gene, and the cell will behave like a normal cell. While the idea is simple, the reality is enormously complicated. Gene therapy has been hyped to such a degree, you might be excused for thinking that it has replaced almost every other type of treatment, or that your local doctor is old-fashioned and not up to date with current treatments if he or she is not prescribing a bottle of genes for you on a regular basis.

Expectations for gene therapy have been unrealistic. More than 600 patients have participated in 100 clinical trials. To date, not one of these trials has been successful. Most authorities now believe that the rush into clinical trials was premature. We do not yet have enough basic science information to launch major clinical trials. While the initial results were disappointing, the scientific and medical community still believe that the long-term prospects for gene therapy are excellent. The United States government now pours $200 million each year into gene therapy. Private industry is estimated to add a similar amount.

Gene therapy works like this. Suppose you have a group of cells with a defective gene—say, for cystic fibrosis (a common inherited disease of the lungs). You take a normal gene from normal cells and insert it into the sick cell by using a harmless virus. Viruses have numerous functional segments. Some of them bind to human cells and allow the virus to get inside the human cell. Once inside, other segments of the viral genes damage the cell. Gene therapists remove the central, undesirable genes from the virus but leave the cell-penetrating segments intact. They splice the desired replacement gene into the virus. The virus can now penetrate the human cell but cannot damage it. Instead the virus transfers the replacement gene to the cell. This type of research is called gene-transfer technology.

Researchers can now transfer genes into many different cell types. A vehicle, such as the virus, for transferring a good gene into cells is called a vector. Different vectors have different advantages and disadvantages. Most are viruses, either retroviruses or adenoviruses. The choice of vector depends on which cells are defective, where they are located, whether they divide frequently, and whether the genes must correct some function in the cell itself or must secrete something that affects other cells. The process is very complicated.

However complicated gene transfer technology may seem, it is only the start of gene "therapy." It is one thing getting a good gene into a cell; it is quite a different story getting it to work properly. We saw in chapter 8 that while structural genes make peptides and proteins, other genes act as promoters or inhibitors switching on and switching off the structural gene in response to various stimuli.

Clinical trials have shown that gene transfer is successful in terms of their scientific purposes. However, they have not yet shown benefit to the patient—gene therapy has not come of age. "Gene therapy is not a failure," says Theodore Friedmann of the University of California – San Diego School of Medicine. "It is simply too immature to deliver yet on its promises." We will have to wait a few more years, or possibly even decades.

Cancer patients will wait even longer. First success will come for those diseases with inherited single-gene defects—diseases such as cystic fibrosis, Duchenne's muscular dystrophy, and hemophilia. Because cancer cells have many gene defects, therapy will be much more complicated. Besides, different cancers have different defects. Even within the same tumor, different cells may have different defects. How will gene therapists identify which ones are critical to replace? Much of the research will be by trial and error. If there is one major gene or group of genes controlling one specific process, they may be able to target the most relevant genes. For example, by replacing the genes responsible for tumor angiogenesis (see chapter 5), they may be able to neutralize metastases. Already trials show that the normal p53 gene can replace aberrant p53 in lung-cancer cells. Other cancer trials are investigating the role of gene therapy in melanoma, brain, breast, liver, and ovarian cancer. The prospects for the future are excellent, but we have a long wait ahead of us.

We can end on another optimistic note. Earlier, we saw that the most important carcinogens are probably in our environment, and we have not yet identified them. While the epidemiology experts continued on their detective detours, public health and cancer agencies launched numerous antismoking campaigns. Their educational and preventive strategies are working. In the United States, age-adjusted cancer mortality increased every year until 1990. Statistics published at the end of 1996 show that in 1991 the trend changed and mortality has continued to decline every year since then. By 1995 the total reduction was 3 percent, and for lung cancer the reduction was almost 4 percent. Other smoking-related cancers also declined. Expressed as percentages, these may seem like small numbers. However, they translate into thousands of saved lives each year. Experts analyzing data argue optimistically that it is possible to cut cancer death rates by 50 percent within the next twenty years. When we identify other important carcinogens, all about us, these figures will improve even more. In the meantime, basic scientists, doctors, and all concerned with cancer will strive to cure or improve the lives of cancer patients. Their dedication, determination, patience, and innovation will ensure success.

Bibliography

Bishop, J.M., and R.A. Weinberg. *Scientific American molecular oncology.* New York: Scientific American Medicine, 1996.

Blan, H.M., and M.L. Springer. Gene therapy—A novel form of drug delivery. *New England Journal of Medicine* 333 (1995):1204–7.

Boguski, M.S., J.H. Olsen, J.D. Boice, Jr., N. Seersholm, A. Bautz, and J.F. Fraumeni, Jr. Hunting for genes in computer data bases. *New England Journal of Medicine* 333, 24 (1995):1594–99.

Folkman, J. Clinical applications of research on angiogenesis. *New England Journal of Medicine* 333, 26 (1995):1757–63.

_____. Fighting cancer by attacking its blood supply. *Scientific American* 275 (1996):116–19.

_____, and C. Murray. Tumor angiogenesis and tissue factor. *Nature Medicine* 2, 2 (1996):167–68.

_____. Tumor dormancy: Not so sleepy after all. *Nature Medicine* 1, 2 (1995):117–18.

Friedmann, T. Human gene therapy—An immature genie, but certainly out of the bottle. *Nature Medicine* 2 (1996):144–47.
Goldenberg, D.M. *Cancer therapy with radio-labeled antibodies.* Boca Raton, Fla.:CRC Press, 1995.
Historic milestones in cancer research. *Seminars in Oncology* 6, 4 (1979):395–541.
Karp, J.E., and S. Broder. Molecular foundations of cancer: New targets for intervention. *Nature Medicine* 1, 4 (1995):309–20.
Linn, S.C., A.H. Honkoop, K. Hoekman, P. Van der Valk, H.M. Pinedo, and G. Giaccone. P53 and Pglycoprotein are often coexpressed and are associated with poor prognosis in breast cancer. *British Journal of Cancer* 74, 1 (1996):63–68.
Marshall, E. A new phase in the war on cancer. *Science* 267, 5203 (1995):1412–15.
McBride, W.H., and G.J. Dougherty. Radiotherapy for genes that cause cancer. *Nature Medicine* 1 (1995):1215–17.
Old, L.J. Immunotherapy and cancer. *Scientific American* 275 (1996):102–9.
Oliff, A., J.B. Gibbs, and F. McCormick. New molecular targets for cancer therapy. *Scientific American* 275 (1996):144–149.
Ruoslahti, E. How cancer spreads. *Scientific American* 275 (1996):42–47.
Sidransky, D. Advances in cancer detection. *Scientific American* 275 (1996):70–75.
Stinchcomb, D.T. Constraining the cell cycle: Regulating cell division and differentiation by gene therapy. *Nature Medicine* 1 (1995):1004–6.
Touchette, N. Gene therapy: Not ready for prime time. *Nature Medicine* 2 (1996):7–8.
Weinberg, R.A. The cell cycle clock and cancer. *Scientific American* 275 (1996): 36–37.
Williams N. An immune boost to the war on cancer. *Science* 272 (1996):28–30.
Williams, R.S. Human gene therapy—Of tortoises and hares. *Nature Medicine* 1 (1995):1137–38.

Appendix: Resources for Cancer Patients and Families

General Cancer Resources

American Cancer Society
1599 Clifton Road N.E.
Atlanta, GA 30329-4251
(800) ACS-2345

National Cancer Institute
9000 Rockville Pike
Bethesda, MD 20892
(800) 4CANCER

Breast Cancer Resources

National Alliance of Breast Cancer Organizations
9 E. 37th Street
New York, NY 10016
(800) 719-9154

National Breast Cancer Coalition
1707 L Street NW
Suite 1060
Washington, DC 20036
(202) 296-7477

Susan G. Komen Foundation
5005 LBJ Freeway
Suite 370
Dallas, TX 75244
(800) IM-AWARE

Y-Me National Organization for Breast Cancer Information and Support
220 W. Van Buren
Chicago, IL 60607
(800) 221-2141

British Organizations Offering Cancer Information and Support

Age Concern England
Astral House
1268 London Road
London SW16 4ER
0181 679 8000

BACUP
3 Bath Place
Rivington Street
London EC2A 3JR
Helpline: 0171 613 2121

Breast Cancer Care
Kiln House
210 New Kings Road
London SW6 4NZ
Helpline: 0171 384 2344
(for UK residents) Freephone: 0808 800 6000
(from outside UK) 0171 384 2365

British Colostomy Association
15 Station Road
Reading
Berks RG1 1LG
01734 391537

Cancer Help Centre
Grove House
Cornwallis Grove
Clifton
Bristol BS8 4PG
01179 743216

Cancer Relief Macmillan Fund
Anchor House
15–19 Britten Street
London SW3 3TZ
0171 351 7811

Cancer Research Campaign
10 Cambridge Terrace
London NW1 4JL
0171 224 1333

Cancerlink
17 Britannia Street
London WC1X 9JN
0171 833 2451

Carers' National Association
20–25 Glasshouse Yard
London EC1A 4JS
0171 490 8898

Citizens Advice Bureau
136–144 City Road
London EC1V 2QN
0171 251 2000

Compassionate Friends
53 North Street
Bristol BS3 1EN
01179 539639

CRUSE—Bereavement Care
126 Sheen Road
Richmond
Surrey TW9 1UR
0181 940 4818

DIAL UK National Association of Disablement and Advice
Park Lodge
St. Catherine's Hospital
Tickhill Road
Doncaster DN4 8QN
01302 310123

Disabled Living Foundation
380 Harrow Road
London W9 2HU
0171 289 6111

Hospice Information Service
St. Christopher's Hospice
51–59 Lawrie Park Road
Sydenham
London SE26 6DZ
0181 778 9252

Imperial Cancer Research Fund
61 Lincoln's Inn Fields
London WC2A 3PX
0171 242 0200

Marie Curie Cancer Care
28 Belgrave Square
London SW1X 8QG
0171 235 3325

Women's National Cancer Control Campaign
Suna House
128–130 Curtain Road
London EC2A 3AR
0171 729 1735

Computerized Search Facilities That Charge for Their Services

The Health Resource
574 Locust Street
Conway, AZ 72032
(800) 949-0090
(501) 329-5272

Planetree Health Resource Center
2040 Webster Street
San Francisco, CA 94115
(415) 923 3680

Schine On-Line Services
39 Brenton Avenue
Providence, RI 02906
(800) 346-3287

World Research Foundation
41 Bell Rock Plaza
Sedona, AZ 86351
(520) 284-3300
email: info@wrf.org

Computer Programs for Searching the Medline Database

Grateful Med
http://igm.nlm.nih.gov/

Health Gate
http://www.healthgate.com/index.shtml

Health World Medline
http://www.healthy.net/library/search/medline.htm

Melcars
http://www.nlm.nih.gov/databases/medlars.html

Paperchase
(800) 722-2075
(617) 278-3900
http://www.mhsource.com/resource/paperchase.html

Silverplatter
Silver Platter Education
246 Walnut St.
Newton, MA 02460-1639
(617) 244-0284
http://www.silverplatter.com/

Medline, the most powerful database in the world, contains more than 8 million references, and most of them come with summaries. Unless you have some experience searching computer databases, looking for information on Medline can be difficult and daunting. A number of software programs can help the user to search the Medline database. Many databases are now free on the Internet. With the exception of Silverplatter, the resources listed above are free. (http://www.ncbi.nlm.nih.gov/PubMed)

Web Sites

Bladder

http://oncolink.upenn.edu/disease/bladder
http://www.cancernews.com/bladder.htm
http://telescan.nk.nl/bladder2.html

Bone Marrow Transplantation

http://oncolink.upenn.edu/specialty/chemo/bmt

Brain

http://oncolink.upenn.edu/disease/brain/
American Brain Tumor Association:
http://neurosurgery.mgh.harvard.edu/abta/

Breast

http://cancer.med.upenn.edu/resources/sites/
http://cancer.med.upenn.edu/disease/breast/
http://nysernet.org/bcic/acs2/pro.ed/index.html/
National Alliance of Breast Cancer Organizations:
http://www.nabco.org/
American Cancer Society:
http://www.cancer.org/bcinfo.html/
Breast cancer genes:
http://oncolink.upenn.edu/resources/brca1/

http://www.homearts.com/depts/chat/promo/49nabc19.htm
http://homearts.com/depts/chat/promo/59nabc19.htm

CHEMOTHERAPY

http://oncolink.upenn.edu/specialty/
http://oncolink.upenn.edu/specialty/surg-onc/
http://oncolink.upenn.edu/specialty/ped-onc/
http://oncolink.upenn.edu/specialty/med-onc/
http://oncolink.upenn.edu/specialty/pain/
http://oncolink.upenn.edu/specialty/rad-onc/
http://oncolink.upenn.edu/specialty/alternative/
http://meds.com/mol/chem-you.html

COLON

http://www.path.jhu.edu/colon/
http://www.path.jhu.edu/rectal/
http://www.path.jhu.edu/anal/
http://www.rattler.cameron.edu/colon/
http://medhlp.netusa.net/general/cancer/lefor.htm

ESOPHAGUS

http://oncolink.upenn.edu/disease/esophageal/

GALLBLADDER

http://oncolink.upenn.edu/disease/gallbladder

KIDNEY

National Kidney Cancer Association:
http://oncolink.upenn.edu/psychosocial/nkcafact.html
http://oncolink.upenn.edu/disease/kidney

LEUKEMIA, LYMPHOMA, AND MYELOMA

Leukemia Society of America:
http://www.leukemia.org/
Adult leukemia:
http://oncolink.upenn.edu/disease/leukemia1/
Lymphoma organizations:
http://www.alumni.Caltech.edu/˜mike/lymphoma/org.html
General lymphoma resources:
http://www.alumni.Caltech.edu/˜mike/lymphoma/general.html
Guide to resources:
http://www.alumni.Caltech.edu/˜mike/lymphoma.html
http://cancer.med.upenn.edu/disease/lymphoma1/
http://oncolink.upenn.edu/disease/nonHodgkins/
http://oncolink.upenn.edu/disease/Hodgkins
http://oncolink.upenn.edu/disease/myeloma/

LIVER

http://oncolink.upenn.edu/disease/liver/

LUNG

http://www.erinet.com/fnadoc/lung.htm
http://www.meds.com/mol/leukemia/lunginfo.html
http://oncolink.upenn.edu/disease/lung1/

OVARY

http://www.cancer.org/ovary.html
http://ovarian.org/m2b/m2b.shtml
http://oncolink.upenn.edu/specialty/gyn-onc/ovarian/

PANCREAS

http://oncolink.upenn.edu/disease/pancreas
http://www.path.jhu.edu/pancreas/

Prostate

American Cancer Society:
http://www.cancer.org/proinfo.html

Sarcomas

http://oncolink.upenn.edu/disease/sarcoma1/

Skin

http://oncolink.upenn.edu/disease/skin1/
Melanoma:
http://oncolink.upenn.edu/disease/melanoma/index.html

Stomach

http://oncolink.upenn.edu/disease/gastric/

Thyroid

http://oncolink.upenn.edu/disease/thyroid/intro-thyroid.html

Uterus and Cervix

http://inforentures.com/cancer/report/v2/crvx1096.html
http://oncolink.upenn.edu/specialty/gyn-onc/endomet/
http://oncolink.upenn.edu/specialty/gyn-onc/cervical/
http://www.cancer.org/cervix.html

Glossary

abl oncogene: An oncogene on chromosome 9. In chronic myeloid leukemia it is translocated onto chromosome 22 and forms a hybrid with another oncogene, *bcr.* The *bcr/abl* gene fusion codes for a protein called p210, which confers a growth advantage to the neoplastic leukemic clone. The *bcr/abl* gene induces leukemia in mice when it is transferred into their nuclei.

bcr oncogene: An oncogene located on chromosome 22. It is important in chronic myeloid leukemia when it translocates with the *abl oncogene* (q.v.)

achalasia: A condition involving the lower portion of the esophagus. The muscle in the involved region is unable to relax properly during peristalsis. The result is a functional obstruction with failure of food to pass properly through the segment. Gradually the remainder of the esophagus near the obstruction becomes distended and food lies within the esophagus for prolonged periods before passing into the stomach. After many years, some patients with this condition develop cancer of the esophagus.

ACTH: Adrenocorticotrophic hormone (q.v.)

adenine: One of the four bases making up the DNA and RNA codes.

adenocarcinoma: A malignant tumor arising from glandular epithelium.

adenoma: A benign tumor arising from glandular epithelial tissue.

adenovirus: This DNA virus infects the upper respiratory tract in normal individuals and causes flu- or hayfever-like symptoms. In immunocompromised victims, it can cause a severe form of pneumonia and be fatal.

adhesion molecule: A chemical that binds cells to each other and also to connective tissue.

adrenal gland: Either of two glands that sit on top of each kidney (one on each). The adrenal is composed of two major zones. The outer zone secretes various corticosteroids such as cortisone. The inner zone (the medulla) secretes epinephrine (adrenaline) and norepinephrine (noradrenaline).

adrenaline: A hormone secreted by the adrenal gland whose function is to control blood pressure and the heart rate. It also contributes to cell metabolism. Also called *epinephrine* (q.v.).

adrenocorticotrophic hormone (ACTH): A hormone secreted from the pituitary gland at the base of the brain that stimulates the adrenal glands to produce corticosteroids. Some tumors, (especially lung cancer) produce ACTH in sufficient quantities to cause *Cushing's syndrome* (q.v.).

AGCT: The four bases that make up the DNA code. The letters stand for adenine, guanine, cytosine, and thymine.

aldosterone: A hormone produced by the adrenal cortex. Its function is to control sodium (salt) metabolism. It is a type of steroid hormone.

allele: One of two or more particular

forms of a gene. One allele may remain inactive while its partner does all the work. Alternatively both alleles may contribute to genetic function. Almost all alleles differ in structure by one or a few bases. Forensic scientists find these differences useful for DNA fingerprinting.

allogeneic BMT: Bone marrow transplantation from a close relative or from somebody with closely matching transplantation genes. The closer the match the less likely that the transplanted cells will be rejected. (c.f. *autologous BMT.*)

amino acid: Small molecules that can link together to form proteins. There are twenty common amino acids, and the way they link to each other and the number of amino acids that are linked together can produce thousands of different proteins with very different properties.

androgen: Male steroid hormone. Some cancers, in particular prostate cancer, grow under the influence of androgens. Sometimes patients with prostate cancer that has metastasized to the spine require removal of the testes in order to remove the androgen effect (surgical castration). Sometimes it is possible to block the affect of androgens using female hormones (stilbestrol) or drugs that reduce the production of testosterone or block its activity.

anemia: Low *hemoglobin* (q.v.). There are many causes. The commonest is iron deficiency.

angiogenesis growth factor: A substance secreted by tumors that induces the surrounding tissue to sprout tiny capillaries, also called tumor angiogenesis growth factor (TAF). New blood vessels are necessary for metastases to occur. They also help deliver blood with its oxygen and nutrients to the tumor cells.

antibody: A special type of protein that binds to target antigens. Antibodies are helpful in eliminating bacteria and other foreign microorganisms. They are also produced in response to antigens present in tumor cells. Antibodies are produced by B-lymphocytes and circulate in the blood and other body fluids. The detection of antibodies specific to tumor antigens may be helpful in diagnosis or in monitoring cancer patients after treatment.

antigen: A molecule, usually a protein, that has the ability to stimulate B-lymphocytes to produce antibodies.

apoptosis: A form of cell death characterized by shrinkage of the cell contents. The cell that has undergone apoptosis is eliminated by macrophages. Apoptosis is a normal physiological process by which the cells are eliminated after they have lived their normal life cycle. The process is controlled by a number of genes; the best known is the *bcl2 oncogene* (q.v.). In many cancers the tumor cells do not undergo apoptosis, and persist indefinitely.

ascites: A collection of fluid in the abdominal peritoneal cavity. There are many benign causes. However, ascites is common when malignant tumors have spread into the peritoneum, such as occurs frequently with ovarian cancer. Small quantities of peritoneal fluid can be detected readily by ultrasound examination.

astrocytes: Specialized cells in the brain and spinal cord. They surround and support the *neurons* (q.v.). Most brain tumors arise from astrocytes and are called astrocytomas.

ataxia: Loss of balance due to poor coordination. Ataxia can result from a large number of disorders affecting the brain or inner ear.

atrophy: The wasting of tissue. Atrophy has many causes, such as inactivity, loss of blood supply, or loss of hormone stimulation.

autologous BMT: Bone marrow transplant in which the patient is his or her own donor. The bone marrow is collected when the patient is in remission, deep-frozen in liquid nitrogen, and returned to the patient after high-dose chemotherapy. (cf. *allogeneic BMT.*)

axilla: The armpit. The axilla contains fat and lymph nodes that are frequently sampled or removed during the surgery for breast cancer. Examination of the lymph nodes helps to determine the stage of the tumor (see *tumor stage*).

B-cell leukemia: Leukemia arising from lymphocytes that immunologically are B lymphocytes (in contrast to T-cells). B-lymphocytes are those cells responsible for the production of circulating antibodies. They are important immune cells.

B symptoms: Systemic symptoms of some cancer patients such as fever, drenching sweats, and weight loss. B symptoms are particularly common in patients with Hodgkin's disease or non-Hodgkin's lymphoma. Whether a patient with lymphoma requires treatment may in some circumstances depend on the presence of B symptoms.

Barrett's esophagus: A change in character of the surface epithelium of the lower esophagus. The lower esophagus is normally lined by squamous epithelium, similar to that in the mouth. In patients with long-standing reflux of gastric acid into the lower esophagus, the surface epithelium becomes like the mucosa lining the stomach or lower intestine. This change is called Barrett's esophagus. Its significance is that it becomes malignant in a small number of patients.

Basal cell carcinoma: One of the commonest of all cancers. It occurs in the skin, commonly on the face. Unlike most cancers, it virtually never metastasizes. However, it continues to grow and destroy tissues locally. When it occurs around the eyelid (a common site) it can cause severe disfigurement and even loss of vision if not removed. Most cancer statistics do not include basal cell carcinomas because they do not metastasize. In this they are like *squamous cell carcinomas* of the skin (q.v.), which rarely metastasize.

base: The chemicals that make up the coding region of the DNA molecule. They are adenine, guanine, cytosine, and thymine.

base pair: The combination of two bases within the DNA molecule. A always combines with T, and C with G.

basement membrane: A protein membrane that separates epithelium from underlying connective tissue. Basement membrane also separates blood vessel endothelial cells from the underlying muscle cells. It provides a temporary barrier to the growth of cancer in epithelial tissues. Cancer confined to cells above the basement membrane is called carcinoma in situ and cannot metastasize until it has broken through the basement membrane.

basophils: Cells that are present in the peripheral blood and bone marrow and are derived from the same cells that produce the neutrophils and eosinophils. Their function is somewhat obscure, but they play a role in some forms of immune reactions. A rise in the number of basophils occurs in *chronic myeloid leukemia* (q.v.).

bcl2 oncogene: A gene that codes for *apoptosis* (q.v.). It is commonly expressed at an abnormally high level in low-grade lymphomas. In some low-grade cancers, cell proliferation can be less than that of normal tissue. However, due to activity of the *bcl2* oncogene, tumor cells persist indefinitely. The cells accumulate and cause the tumor to grow.

Beckwith-Wiedemann syndrome: A genetic disorder characterized by overgrowth of many tissues. Structural abnormalities occur within the kidney and these predispose to the development of Wilms' tumor. Wilms' tumor is one of the commonest tumors of infancy and usually occurs sporadically (that is, with no genetic predisposition).

benign neoplasm: A new growth or tumor that does not invade and destroy normal tissues or metastasize. It can be composed of epithelial tissue or stroma (such as muscle). However, it can cause symptoms by local pressure on surrounding tissues. For example, in the uterus it may cause bleeding from the surface of the endometrium. If benign neoplasms arise in an endocrine gland, they sometimes are functionally active—they may produce the same hormone as the tissue from which they arise. Benign tumors rarely become malignant. However, some, such as adenomas/polyps in the intestine, may evolve into malignancy over a period of many years.

benign prostatic hyperplasia: An enlargement of the prostate gland that may obstruct urination. Treatment is usually surgical removal of the obstructing tissue with the aid of an endoscope. More recently, certain medications have been successful in shrinking the prostate gland.

biopsy: Removal of a piece of tissue for microscopic examination. A biopsy may be a tiny fragment (less than 1mm) removed through a needle or it may be a large excision. Many biopsies remove just a sample of tissue 2–3mm in size for initial diagnostic purposes. In addition to making a diagnosis, the pathologist can often grade the tumor on the basis of the biopsy. Sometimes—for example, with a breast lump—the biopsy procedure may be therapeutic, as the entire lesion may be removed by the biopsy procedure.

blast: Immature white blood cell or immune cell (lymphocyte). Blasts are primitive cells characteristic of acute leukemias or high-grade lymphomas.

Bloom's syndrome: A rare genetic disorder in which the skin is especially sensitive to sunlight. Patients are at greater risk for leukemia than the general population.

bone marrow: Soft spongy tissue residing within the bone marrow spaces. The cells composing this tissue give rise to circulating blood cells—red blood cells, white blood cells, and platelets.

bone marrow transplant (BMT): Replacement of a patient's depleted bone marrow with healthy marrow cells from a donor. Depletion usually results from chemotherapy and leaves the patient prone to overwhelming infection with a high risk of death. The bone marrow comes either from the patient himself or herself or from someone with closely related genes (usually someone from the same family).

brachytherapy: A form of radiation therapy wherein radioactive particles are embedded directly into the tissue (as distinct from external beam radiation).

BRCA1 and BRCA2: Genes with diagnostic significance for certain hereditary cancers. Approximately 10 percent of breast cancers are familial and are due to hereditary genetic mutations. Those that have been identified to date are mostly in the genes known as BRCA1 and BRCA2. Women with mutations in these genes have a high incidence of breast cancer and also ovarian cancer. The precise function of BRCA1 and BRCA2 under normal circumstances is not known.

bronchoscope: An optical instrument for inspecting the insides of the bronchi in the lungs. The instrument contains a small biopsy forceps for sampling tumor tissue. It can also be used to introduce a fine biopsy needle through the bronchial wall into adjacent lung tissue.

Burkitt's lymphoma: A high-grade, rapidly proliferating cancer of B-lymphocytes. In Africa it has a strong association with the Epstein-Barr virus.

CA-125: An antigen present in the circulating blood of patients with ovarian cancer and some other forms of cancer. The level of CA-125 in the blood roughly parallels the amount of tumor present. When the primary tumor has been treated, CA-125 levels drop to normal. If cancer recurs, levels increase again in the peripheral blood. Monitoring CA-125 helps detect early recurrence.

cachexia: Severe generalized wasting. Cachexia is common in patients with terminal cancer and AIDS. Other diseases can also cause cachexia. (See also *tumor necrosis factor.*)

cancer: Any form of malignancy.

carcinogen: A substance that can cause cancer. (See also *chemical carcinogen.*)

carcinoma: A malignant tumor arising from epithelial tissue. Most adult cancers are carcinomas.

carcinoma in situ: The early phase of malignant epithelial tumors, which is confined above a basement membrane. Carcinoma in situ cannot metastasize until it has transformed into an invasive carcinoma and has penetrated the basement membrane. Carcinoma in situ is commonly seen in the skin, breast, cervix, and intestine.

carcinosarcoma: A malignant tumor composed of two malignant tissues. One of these is epithelial-derived and the other is from connective tissue. Carcinosarcomas are rare.

case control study: A form of scientific investigation in which a group of patients with a certain medical problem—for example, breast cancer—is compared to a group of people who do not have that medical problem. The two groups are selected for their similarity in age, sex, and many other variables. They are studied to determine what factors (such as cigarette smoking or living in a certain location) might be linked with the disease. This is a form of epidemiological study.

castration: Surgical removal of the testes. For some patients with metastatic prostatic cancer castration can relieve bone pain by abolishing their active androgen hormones. Alternatively, in some patients the same effects can be produced by medication.

catecholamines: A group of chemically related substances produced by the body. Of significance are norepinephrine and epinephrine, which are released from the adrenal medulla. Among their functions are maintaining tone in the muscle of blood vessels and contributing to the heart rate. Tumors arising from the adrenal medulla increase the amount of catecholamines in the blood. Neuroblastoma in children (q.v.) is a form of cancer that arises from the cells in the adrenal medulla. In adults, pheochromocytomas (q.v.) also arise from adrenal medulla cells.

CD34: A marker antigen present on the surface of certain cell types. In particular it is found on the surface of bone-marrow stem cells and stem cells circulating in the peripheral blood. This marker can be used to identify and quantify the number of circulating stem cells for the purpose of stem cell transplantation.

cell: The smallest complete independent structure of a tissue or organ. The cell is the basic functional unit of all living tissue. Each cell is composed of an outer cell membrane and an inner bag of fluid, enzymes, and proteins. The nucleus resides within the cell as a separate membrane-bound structure and is surrounded by *cytoplasm* (q.v.). Chromosomes and genetic material are contained within the nucleus. The cell's metabolism is directed by *organelles* (q.v.) present in the cytoplasm.

cell cycle: The progression of phases in the life of a cell, such as *G0, G1, S, G2,* and *M* (q.v.). Most cells grow and divide and form new daughter cells. This process of cell proliferation is controlled by a large number of genes. Some cells have a rapid cell cycle, such as bone marrow cells, cells lining the skin, and cells lining the intestine. Some cells, such as neurons, do not divide. Other cells proliferate when injured or stimulated. Tumor cells have very abnormal cell cycles.

centromere: A tight constriction separating the long and short arms of chromosome pairs.

CGL: Chronic granulocytic leukemia. (See *chronic myeloid leukemia.*)

chemical carcinogen: A cancer-producing chemical such as asbestos, the tars and chemicals in cigarette smoke, and polyvinyl chloride.

chemotherapy: Treatment for cancer that involves primarily the use of drugs (as distinct from surgery and radiation therapy).

chondrosarcoma: A malignant tumor of cartilage, usually arising in bone.

chromosomal rearrangements: Movement of large DNA segments or fragments of chromosomes from one part of a chromosome to another part. Such rearrangements may alter cell function.

chromosome: The gene-carrying component of cells that determines hereditary characteristics. Each cell contains 46 chromosomes. Each chromosome consists of a complex, compactly folded strand of DNA. The DNA is wound around a protein core. Half of the genetic material is derived from each parent. When a cell divides, its chromosomes split and reduplicate, with an equal amount of DNA going into each of the daughter cells.

chronic granulocytic leukemia (GGL): Another name for *chronic myeloid leukemia* (q.v.).

chronic lymphocytic leukemia (chronic lymphatic leukemia or CLL): A low-grade leukemia of adults. Even without treatment, prolonged survival is often possible.

chronic myeloid leukemia (CML): A common form of malignancy of the white blood cells in adults. The tumor is derived from the neutrophils or granulocytes in the bone marrow.

cilia: Tiny filamentous structures on the surface of some lining epithelial cells, in particular those lining the bronchi in the lungs. Cilia are motile and propel fluid, mucus, and particles along the surface of the cells.

cirrhosis: A disease of the liver characterized by chronic inflammation, and replacement of the normal structure of the liver by fibrous tissue and small nodules of regenerating liver cells. There are many causes of cirrhosis. The commonest is alcohol abuse. In certain parts of the world hepatitis B is the commonest cause. In some patients the regenerative cells eventually transform into a malignant tumor (hepatocellular carcinoma, also known as hepatoma).

clinical trial: A scientific epidemiological investigation carried out under rigorous conditions to compare the value and complications of one particular type of treatment with another. Often neither the doctors nor the patients know which treatment they are receiving (a kind of trial known as a double blind trial).

CLL: See *chronic lymphatic leukemia.*

clone: A group of cells all derived from one single cell. Most cancers are thought to be monoclonal in origin. Tumors frequently have subclones with different characteristics and biological advantages.

clustering: Multiple occurrences of one form of cancer within a readily definable population of patients. For example, leukemia may affect three or four children in the same small village or town. While clustering frequently gives rise to some form of investigation, the vast majority of clusters eventually are explained by random statistical variation.

CML: See *chronic myeloid leukemia.*

codon: A sequence of three complex chemicals in the cell that serve as codes to direct the production of amino acids. Sixty-one codes are translated into twenty amino acids. Between one and six codons account for each amino acid. Three codons function as stop signals that indicate that the end of the protein has been reached.

cohort study: A scientific epidemiological study in which a large population (say 100,000) are questioned in detail about their habits and their environment. The population is then followed for a number of years or decades to see who gets sick and who does not. Researchers analyze the data and identify what factors might account for the difference between those who get sick and those who do not.

colectomy: Surgical removal of the colon, in part or in total.

colonoscope: An optical instrument for visualizing the inside of the colon and its mucosal lining. Lesions can be biopsied through the colonoscope.

colostomy: An opening onto the outer wall of the abdomen with which the colon can communicate directly. A colostomy may be necessary as a temporary procedure with certain forms of colonic surgery. For patients with cancers located at the distal end of the rectum, the surgery required to remove the tumor may leave the patient with a permanent colostomy.

columnar cells: Epithelial cells lining the surface of many tissues. They are called columnar because they have a tall columnar appearance.

congenital: Present at birth. Some congenital abnormalities are not hereditary but are due to some damaging effect on the fetus during pregnancy.

congenital immunodeficiency: Immunodeficiency present at birth. Congenital immunodeficiency is usually hereditary. Patients with immunodeficiency of any type are more prone to get cancer.

connective tissue: A loose permeative substance composed of cells, water, proteins, and other chemicals that surrounds and binds together muscles, nerves, blood vessels, and all tissues in all organs. It is also known as stroma.

cortisol: A steroid hormone produced by the adrenal cortex. It has strong anti-inflammatory properties. Excess therapeutic administration or overproduction causes Cushing's syndrome.

craniopharyngioma: A benign tumor arising at the base of the brain just above the pituitary gland. Although craniopharyngioma is benign, it can infiltrate the surrounding brain and destroy the pituitary, and it may be difficult to remove. For most patients the treatment is surgical.

CT (computerized tomography) scan: A type of X-ray that allows the study of the inside of the body in great detail.

curative treatment: Treatment aimed at achieving a complete cure.

Cushing's syndrome: A condition caused by excess cortisol or cortisol-like hormones characterized by obesity, osteoporosis, fragile skin, and often high blood pressure.

cyst: A lump or bump composed of fluid with a surrounding thin wall. Sometimes a cyst is congenital or due to an obstructive secretion. At other times it is caused by a benign or malignant tumor in which the cells lining the wall of the cyst are neoplastic.

cystic teratoma: See *teratoma.*

cystoscope: An optical instrument for visualizing the inside of the urinary bladder. Biopsies may be taken through the cystoscope.

cytochemical profile: An analysis of the chemical constituents of a cell. Often it is possible to produce a microscopic picture by visualizing profiles of these chemicals. Such profiles may be helpful in distinguishing one type of leukemia from another. Cytochemical tests are carried out on aspirated bone marrow cells or on blood cells. A similar procedure can be performed on tissue sections, a technique known as histochemistry.

cytogenetics: The study of genetic abnormalities by examining chromosome preparations.

cytokine: A chemical released by many types of cell, especially immune and inflammatory cells. Different cytokines have different actions. In general, they modify the behavior of other cells.

cytologist: A paramedic specially trained to identify malignant and premalignant changes in cytology preparations, such as cervical cytology smears.

cytology: The microscopic study of cellular abnormalities in preparations that were made by smearing cells onto a glass slide. It differs from histology in that entire cells or groups of cells are examined but little or no tissue architecture is present. In contrast, histology preparations show microarchitecture. Because histology preparations show cells growing in relation to each other and also in relationship to basement membrane and stroma, histologic appearances tend to be more definitive than cytology. See also *diagnostic cytology, screening cytology.*

cytoplasm: That portion of the cell surrounding the nucleus and surrounded by the cell membrane. It contains mitochondria, ribosomes, endoplasmic reticulum, water, proteins, and chemicals. Most protein, carbohydrate, and fat production takes place in the cytoplasm.

cytosine: One of the four bases making up the DNA code.

DCIS: See *ductal carcinoma.*

debulk: The surgical removal of part of a tumor. The purpose of cancer surgery is to remove the cancer entirely with some surrounding normal tissue. Sometimes it is not possible to do this. In such circumstances it may be beneficial to remove a large portion or most of the tumor. The remaining tumor sometimes responds to radiotherapy or chemotherapy.

dementia: An acquired, persistent impairment of mental function, which affects language, memory, emotion and cognition. There are many causes, Alzheimer's being the commonest. It also occurs in some patients with AIDS and cancer.

deoxyribose: The sugar molecule that makes up the outer structure of the DNA helix.

dermis: That portion of the skin just beneath the surface.

dermoid cyst: A benign cystic tumor of the ovary composed of a mixture of mature adult tissues. About 10 percent of all ovarian tumors are dermoid cysts, also known as benign cystic *teratomas* (q.v.).

desmosome: Velcro-like connections that bind epithelial cells together. Desmosomes can be studied with the electron microscope. They are poorly formed in cancer cells. Consequently, malignant cells are bound together loosely.

diagnostic cytology: The microscopic study of cells removed from a visible abnormality. If the lesion is deep within the body, it may be localized by radiological procedures. In such circumstances a fine needle is introduced into the abnormality and cells are aspirated. (see *fine needle aspiration cytology.*) *Screening cytology* (q.v.) is the term used to describe the examination of cells that are removed from a normal person, as part of a screening procedure rather than directly from a visible lesion.

diethylstilbestrol: A female hormone similar to estrogen. An unusual form of adenocarcinoma occurring in the vaginas of young females has been linked to the administration of this drug to their mothers during pregnancy.

differentiation: The process wherein normal cells and tissue mature toward their final appearance, e.g., as brain, heart, or liver cells. In cancer it refers to the process wherein the tumor tissue tries to simulate as closely as possible the tissue from which it arose. The term *well-differentiated* means that the tumor closely resembles normal tissue. Poorly differentiated tumors do not bear a close resemblance to the tissue they originated from. The term *undifferentiated* refers to a tumor with a primitive embryonic appearance bearing no resemblance to any normal tissue.

DNA: Deoxyribonucleic acid—a molecule with a double helix configuration responsible for storing and passing on genetic information. All genes are made from DNA.

DNA code: The sequence of bases

(arranged in groups of three or triplets) that code for a particular amino acid. A group of triplets code for a peptide or a protein.

DNA virus: A virus consisting of a core of DNA surrounded by a protein coat. Most disease-causing viruses are DNA viruses. A smaller number of viruses are classified as RNA viruses. A typical example is the AIDS retrovirus.

ductal carcinoma: The commonest type of breast cancer. It may be in situ, that is, confined to the epithelium lining the breast ducts (ductal carcinoma in situ). More commonly it is invasive and called invasive ductal carcinoma.

Duke's staging system: A term used to classify the extent of spread (the stage) of a tumor. The least amount of spread is when it is confined to the mucosa in colonic cancers (Dukes A). Dukes B means that the tumor has invaded the muscle wall of the intestine. Dukes C means that the draining lymph nodes have become involved. Dukes D means that the cancer has spread to the liver. Prognosis correlates relatively closely with the extent of spread. Patients with Dukes A stage have approximately 90 percent five-year survival (and almost all these patients are cured). Only a very small percentage of patients whose tumor has spread to the liver at the time of diagnosis survive beyond five years.

dysphagia: Difficulty in swallowing. Patients often have the sensation that food sticks behind their breastbone and moves slowly downward. Dysphagia is commonly due to a narrowing of the esophagus. If the narrowing continues, as happens with progressive tumor growth, dysphagia gets increasingly worse. Eventually patients may be able to swallow only fluid.

dysplasia: A premalignant microscopic change characterised by enlarged, irregular nuclei. There are varying degrees of dysplasia. The most severe progress to carcinoma in situ and invasive carcinoma. Others revert to normal.

Ectoderm: The embryonic layer that contributes primarily to the skin, breasts, and nervous system (brain and spinal cord). Cf. *endoderm, mesoderm.*

embryo: The stage of growth between the time an egg is fertilized until approximately the seventh or eighth week of pregnancy. During this time there is rapid growth and differentiation of all major organ systems. Cf. *fetus.*

emphysema: A generalized condition of the lung in which there is overdistention of the terminal airways with destruction of lung tissue. Usually it is associated with chronic bronchitis. Cigarette smoking is the main cause.

endoderm: The embryonic layer that contributes primarily to the lung and intestine. Cf. *ectoderm, mesoderm.*

endometrium: The lining of the uterus (womb), which is shed at the time of menstruation. Each month the new layer of endometrium is grown and shed. Endometrial cancer usually arises after menopause, from the glands within the endometrium. It is an adenocarcinoma.

endoplasmic reticulum: A network of membranes and tubes present throughout the cytoplasm of every cell. There are two major forms. The rough endoplasmic reticulum has numerous ribosomes bound to the surface, and they are responsible for producing proteins. The smooth endoplasmic reticulum is responsible primarily for the synthesis of fats (lipids).

endoscope: An optical instrument (usually made of fiber optics) for looking inside a body cavity or hollow organ.

enzyme: A protein that speeds up chemical reactions in tissues. Enzymes may act within the cell to speed up the synthesis of molecules. However, enzymes are also secreted from the cell into their surrounding environment, where they may help to break down unwanted tissue. They are also secreted into the intestine to speed up digestion.

eosinophil: A form of white blood cell

(leukocyte). Eosinophils make up approximately 1–3 percent of all white blood cells. They contain proteins within the cytoplasm that participate in allergic immune reactions. A rise in eosinophil levels is common in patients with allergies and parasite infections. Eosinophil levels also rise in patients with chronic myeloid leukemia.

epidemiology: The scientific study of how disease affects large populations, rather than individuals. Epidemiology uses biostatistics as its main tool to investigate the association between illness and possible causes. By identifying associations, epidemiologists may provide clues about the cause of a specific disease. However, it does not provide proof. Methods other than observation and association are required for proof of causation. Epidemiological studies are either *descriptive* or *analytic*. Descriptive studies determine the nature of the population affected by a specific disease, taking into account such factors as age, sex, ethnic origin, and occupation. Descriptive studies may identify new diseases or suggest a previously unrecognized association between a risk factor and a disease. Analytic studies test the conclusions drawn from descriptive surveys, or from laboratory observations. *Case control studies* and *cohort studies* (q.v.) are forms of analytic epidemiological studies. The results of epidemiological studies may be used to plan new health services, such as cancer screening, or to evaluate the overall health of a given population.

epidermis: The outer layer of the skin (that part of the skin that you can see).

epinephrine: A hormone that is released from the cells and the adrenal medulla (also known as adrenaline). It and its closely related cousin norepinephrine stimulate the heart to beat more quickly. It has a rapid and transient effect on many other tissues, in particular smooth muscle cells in the walls of blood vessels and the intestine. Epinephrine and norepinephrine are released in excessive amounts from a benign tumor of the adrenal gland called a pheochromocytoma. The rise in these hormones causes high blood pressure, headache, sweating, nausea, vomiting, and fainting spells. It may cause sudden death by disturbing heart rhythm.

epithelium: The covering or lining of organs. For example, the outer layer of the skin and the inner layers of lungs, intestinal tract, urinary tract, uterus, vagina, and various ducts are all lined by epithelium.

Epstein-Barr virus (EBV): A virus that commonly causes infectious mononucleosis (glandular fever). However, there is a strong association between it and a number of cancers. The association is strongest in cancer arising in the back of the throat in China and with Burkitt's lymphoma in Central Africa.

erythrocytes: Also known as red blood cells. Erythrocytes are the oxygen-carrying cells of the body. They contain large amounts of hemoglobin. This protein binds oxygen from the inhaled air in the lungs. Erythrocytes in the blood circulate to all tissues, where hemoglobin releases oxygen. Erythroblasts are the precursor cells of erythrocytes. An exceptionally rare form of leukemia arises from these cells and is called erythroblastic leukemia (also known as diGuglielmo's disease).

exon: The exons are those segments of a gene that are responsible for DNA coding. They are, as it were, the active parts of the gene. Exons are separated by noncoding segments called introns. During the process of coding and the formation of messenger RNA, the introns are spliced away, leaving the active component coded in the messenger *RNA* (q.v.).

FAB: French, American, British classification of acute leukemia. FAB is based primarily on the microscopic appearance of the cells.

false negative diagnosis: The conclusion that a patient does not have a particular disease, when in reality the patient has the disease. False negatives are relatively rare when a combination of methods or tests is used before arriving at a final diagnosis. However, it is not uncommon for a single test to have a false negative result. Sometimes, especially in the early stages of the disease, some tests may be positive and some tests may be negative, and the physician ends up with an inconclusive result. In such a case the diagnostic process is put on temporary hold. After a period of time (often months) the tests are repeated. Usually the correct diagnosis becomes apparent after a period of time and observation.

false positive diagnosis: The conclusion that a patient has a particular disease, when in reality the patient does not have the disease. False positives are even less common than false negative diagnoses.

familial adenomatosis polyposis (FAP): A hereditary condition characterized by the presence of dozens to thousands of polyps throughout the colon. Such polyps are premalignant and arise from a genetic mutation on chromosome 5. Colectomy is the treatment of choice and prevents the onset of cancer.

Fanconi's anemia: A hereditary form of anemia in which the patient is prone to develop leukemia.

fetus: The stage in human development that follows the embryonic period, usually from the eighth week after fertilization until birth. Cf. *embryo.*

FHIT gene: A suppressor gene responsible for altering DNA synthesis and cell division. It is located at a fragile site and is altered in many cancers.

fibroadenoma: A benign tumor of the breast composed of a mixture of epithelium and connective tissue.

fibrocystic disease (change): A benign condition of the breast characterized by the presence of cysts, increased glandular proliferation, and increased fibrous tissue. Its importance is that it produces a lump that must be distinguished from cancer.

fibroid: A benign tumor of the muscular part of the uterus (See also *leiomyoma*).

fibrous tissue: Dense connective tissue composed of collagen and other similar proteins, without epithelial components.

fine needle aspiration cytology (FNAC): A technique for removing a tiny number of cells through a fine-bore needle. Its main advantage is that it can get a sample of the cells from deeply located lesions without surgery. The needle is inserted into the lesion. If the lesion is superficial or palpable, the procedure can be carried out by a surgeon, pathologist, or physician trained to carry out the technique. If the lesion is deep within the lung, pancreas, or some other internal organ, the procedure is usually carried out by a radiologist under CT or ultrasound guidance. The disadvantage of the technique is that it has a moderately high false negative result (the number of false negatives depends on the lesion being sampled) and the specimen provided is, in general, inferior to a tissue biopsy. However, it is often a safe, efficient, and cost-effective method of obtaining a rapid diagnosis.

five-year survival rate: The percentage of patients projected to live at least five years longer. The term is commonly used to evaluate response to treatment and prognosis. Usually patients who survive for five years, with no evidence of recurrent disease, are cured. Some cancers, however, recur even after five years. The term does not equate with absolute cure.

fragile sites: Locations on chromosomes that are particularly susceptible to mutation or break points for translocations. They are frequently found at the sites of oncogene activation.

French, American, British Classification: see FAB

G0: The resting phase of the cell cycle.

G1: The first gap phase of the cell cycle.

G2: The second gap phase of the cell cycle.

gastroscope: An optical instrument for examining the inside of the stomach. It is also used to examine the esophagus and duodenum.

GCSF: (See granulocyte colony stimulating factor.)

gene: Those fragments of DNA that code for a specific chemical product (e.g., a protein) or human characteristic.

gene therapy: A form of treatment in which a defective gene is replaced by a normal gene. Gene therapy for cancer is still at the experimental stage.

glandular mucosa: Epithelial lining, such as occurs throughout the gastrointestinal tract, characterized by the presence of numerous glands that secrete various fluids and enzymes onto the surface of the mucosa.

Gleason grading system: A histopathological grading for prostate cancer. The Gleason system is relatively accurate in predicting which tumors will behave aggressively and are likely to metastasize.

glioma: A primary brain tumor. Most gliomas arise from *astrocytes* (q.v.). Gliomas are malignant and vary from slow-growing low-grade tumors to rapidly growing high-grade tumors.

grade: The degree of malignancy as determined by microscopic examination. There are many grading systems. Most cancers can be divided into low, intermediate, and high grades. In general, low-grade tumors grow slowly and are biologically less aggressive than high-grade tumors. Low-grade tumors tend to be more amenable to surgical removal, metastasize later, and do not respond well to chemotherapy. There are many exceptions to these generalizations.

graft versus host disease: A condition that arises when grafted tissue launches an immune-attack on its host. After bone marrow transplantation, for example, from another individual (allogeneic graft), the grafted lymphocytes in the bone marrow proliferate and launch an immunological reaction against host tissue. The result of this attack is seen most commonly in the skin and gastrointestinal tract.

granulocyte: A circulating white blood cell with strong bacteria-fighting properties. Granulocytes are also called neutrophils and are the commonest white cells in the circulating blood. During chemotherapy some patients lose bone marrow function. The number of circulating granulocytes (neutrophils) may become so low that the patient requires a granulocyte transfusion to prevent overwhelming infection.

granulocyte colony stimulating factor (GCSF): A chemical that stimulates the neutrophils or granulocytes in the bone marrow to proliferate and move into the peripheral blood. GCSF has been cloned and is now produced in injectable form (like insulin). It is invaluable for patients with low white cell counts when their marrow is suppressed from chemotherapy. It prevents such patients from getting overwhelming infections.

guanine: One of the four bases that make up the DNA code.

Helicobacter pylori: A tiny microorganism thought to be largely responsible for gastritis and peptic ulceration of the stomach and duodenum. Recently, it has been implicated as a possible cause or cofactor in gastric carcinoma and gastric lymphoma.

helix: A coiled, spiral-like structure found in many molecules, including DNA.

hematologist: A medically qualified doctor specializing in the treatment of patients with various blood diseases, such as leukemia.

hematoxylin: A dye used by cytologists and histopathologists to stain the cell nucleus so that it can be examined microscopically.

hemoglobin: The oxygen-carrying protein present in the red blood cells.

hemoptysis: Coughing up blood. There are many causes of hemoptysis other than lung cancer.

hereditary: A condition or characteristic inherited from one's parents or grandparents.

hereditary nonpolyposis colon cancer (HNPCC): A type of colon cancer due to mutations in DNA repair genes. Up to 10 percent of all colon cancers may be due to this condition. It usually affects patients in their mid 40s. It is also known as the Lynch syndrome.

histology: See *cytology, diagnostic cytology,* and *screening cytology.*

histopathology: The microscopic study of disease.

Hodgkin's disease: A form of lymphoma characterized by the presence of distinctive tumor cells known as Reed-Sternberg cells. It involves lymph nodes in any area of the body and can eventually spread to bone marrow, liver, and other organs. It is highly sensitive to chemotherapy and radiotherapy and treatment is curative for most patients.

homeobox genes: Genes responsible for differentiation of tissues and organs in the embryo. Mutation in homeobox genes may be responsible for loss of differentiation in malignant tumors.

hormone: A chemical released from one tissue that passes through the circulation and exerts its influence on a distant tissue. Typical examples are insulin, growth hormone, and epinephrine.

HPV: See *human papilloma virus.*

HTLV (human T cell lymphotrophic virus): A group of retroviruses, some of which are responsible for AIDS and for an uncommon form of leukemia.

human papilloma virus (HPV): A virus that infects many human tissues and is thought to be a major factor in the initiation and progression of cervical cancer. HPV have many different subtypes, and some are more carcinogenic then others. It appears that HPV requires the presence of other factors in combination in order to be carcinogenic.

hyperplasia: An increase in the number of cells in any tissue. The extra cells may cause tissue enlargement, as in benign prostatic hyperplasia.

hypertrophy: An increase in the size of a tissue or organ due to an increase in the size of individual cells.

hysterectomy: Surgical removal of the uterus.

immune cells: Cells responsible for immunological reactions. The two types are T and B cells (lymphocytes). Macrophages also play a role in the immunological system by processing information for the T and B cells.

immunoglobulin: A form of protein present in blood and tissues. It is the main constituent of antibodies and is produced by B cells.

immunotherapy: A form of therapy designed to enhance the body's immune system against disease. In relation to cancer, it attempts to trick immune cells into reacting to cancer cells as foreign cells and rejecting them, as they would an organ transplant.

intron: Piece of genetic material that lies between exons. Introns are noncoding portions of DNA. Until recently they were thought to have no significant function. Some introns may have a controlling effect on the coding segments of DNA (exons). Their precise function is poorly understood.

junk DNA: The large portion of the genetic material in each cell that appears to have no useful function. Much of this DNA consists of introns. It is likely that much of it has functions that we do not yet understand.

Kaposi's sarcoma: A malignant tumor arising from the endothelial cells that line tiny capillaries. This commonly occurs in patients with AIDS. It is often multifocal. Usually the skin has multiple blackish nodules. However, it can involve any tissue in the body.

karyotype: A photographic rearrangement of chromosomes showing each pair in sequence, from chromosome 1 to chromosome 23. The purpose of the karyotype is to examine the microscopic structure of each chromosome.

labile cells: Cells such as those of the bone marrow and epithelial cells lining the intestine and skin. Labile cells proliferate and multiply rapidly—usually every few days, but if necessary within hours. Cf. *permanent cells, stable cells.*

laparotomy: A surgical procedure to inspect or remove diseased tissue within the abdomen. More recently many of the procedures requiring laparotomy can be performed through a specially designed *endoscope* (q.v.). This is termed endoscopic laparotomy.

leiomyoma: A benign smooth-muscle tumor. Leiomyomas can occur in virtually any tissue in the body. Most commonly they are found in the wall of the uterus, where they are called fibroids.

leiomyosarcoma: A type of cancer composed of malignant smooth-muscle cells. Smooth-muscle cells are present in the wall of the intestine, the uterus, and many other tissues.

leukemia: Cancer of the blood-forming cells in the bone marrow. There are many varieties, each derived from a specific type of white blood cell.

Li-Fraumeni syndrome: A rare disorder characterized by the presence of many different cancers in the same individual. It is due to an inherited mutation of the *p53 oncogene* (q.v.).

limb-sparing surgery: A type of surgery performed for bone cancer, as an alternative to amputation. The tumor and a segment of adjacent bone is removed and replaced by a metal prosthesis. In rare circumstances it may be possible to induce the original bone to regenerate, thus avoiding the necessity for prosthesis.

lobular carcinoma: A type of breast cancer arising from the lobular epithelium. Infiltrating lobular carcinoma is one of the two commoner breast cancers (the other is infiltrating ductal carcinoma).

local spread (or local invasion): Spread to adjacent tissues. For example, cancer of the thyroid gland spreads through the thyroid into the surrounding connective tissue in the neck.

lumpectomy: A term commonly applied to a surgical procedure to remove a tumor with minimal surrounding normal tissue. Breast cancers are frequently removed by lumpectomy.

lymph nodes: Small collections of lymphocytes and macrophages, bound together like a pea pod. Lymphatic channels lead into and out from each lymph node. There are hundreds of lymph nodes scattered throughout the body. They are the main tissues of the immune system. Within lymph nodes T and B cells proliferate in response to an immunological insult.

lymphatics: The tiny threadlike channels carrying fluid into, and from, lymph nodes. Within the lymphatic fluid lymphocytes travel to and from lymph nodes. Lymphocytes and their lymph nodes monitor every tissue in the body.

lymphoblast: An immature primitive lymphocyte. Lymphocytes transform into lymphoblasts in response to immune stimulation. Lymphoblasts are also the neoplastic cells in acute lymphatic leukemia.

lymphocyte: The cells controlling the immune system. They are classified as T lymphocytes and B lymphocytes. Lymphatic and lymphoblastic leukemias arise from lymphocytes, as do non-Hodgkin's lymphomas.

lymphoma: See *malignant lymphoma.*

Lynch syndrome: See *hereditary monpolyposis colon cancer.*

Lysosome: An organelle (q.v.) in the cytoplasm of many cells that contains collections of digestive enzymes and is particularly abundant in neutrophils and macrophages. In these cells they contribute to the destruction of ingested foreign material or bacteria.

M phase: The mitotic phase of the cell cycle during which cells divide to form two daughter cells.

macrophage: A cell present in all tissues and in the blood whose function is to digest foreign material (including bacteria) or dead tissue. They also interact with lymphocytes to participate in the immune response.

malignant lymphoma: A malignant tumor arising from lymphoid tissue in lymph nodes and other tissues. Lymphomas are classified into two main groups—*non-Hodgkin's lymphomas* (q.v.) and *Hodgkin's disease* (q.v.). Each of these has many subclassifications.

malignant melanoma: A highly aggressive malignant tumor arising from the melanocytes (pigment-producing) cells of the skin. Although melanoma is highly aggressive, it can be cured if diagnosed and removed at an early stage. Rarely, malignant melanomas arise in tissues other than skin.

mammography: A special X-ray of the breasts, used to identify and locate breast cancer. Its main advantage is that it can detect carcinoma in situ (q.v.) or very small infiltrating carcinomas too small to be clinically palpable.

mastectomy: Surgical removal of the breast. A simple mastectomy removes the breast and overlying skin but no underlying deep tissues. A radical mastectomy removes the breast with underlying muscle, connective tissue, and axillary (armpit) contents. Radical mastectomies are rarely performed now, as less radical surgical procedures achieve the same effect and are less mutilating.

medline: An electronic database containing the names of all important published articles in the medical literature, including a summary of most articles.

megakaryocyte: Precursor cell in the bone marrow that produces platelets (necessary to prevent bleeding).

meiosis: A form of cell division confined to germ cells (sperm cells in the testes and ova in the ovaries). During the process of meiosis each resulting cell has half the normal number of chromosomes.

melanin: Brown or blackish pigment present in the skin.

melanocytes: Pigment-containing cells in the lower portion of the epidermis in the skin. Benign tumors arising from melanocytes are called *nevi* (see *nevus*). Malignant tumors are called *melanomas* (see *malignant melanoma*).

melanoma: See *malignant melanoma.*

mesenchyme: Loose connective tissue present throughout the body. It has the same meaning as the term *soft tissue* and arises from the embryonic mesoderm. It helps to bind other tissues and organs together. However, it has a broader meaning than soft tissue, in that smooth muscle and some other important tissues arise from mesenchyme. Malignant tumors arising from mesenchyme are *sarcomas* (q.v.).

mesoderm: The embryonic layer that gives rise to muscle, bone, bone marrow, immune cells and much of the connective tissue throughout the body. Cf. *ectoderm, endoderm.*

messenger RNA: See *mRNA.*

metastases: Spread of tumor from one site to another. For instance, cancer of the colon metastasizes to draining lymph nodes and also to the liver. The common routes for metastases are the lymphatics and bloodstream.

micrometastases: Metastases consisting of one or a few cells. They may be too small to be detected by routine light microscopy. However, more sensitive molecular biology techniques can detect many forms of micrometastases. The clinical significance of micrometastases is not yet clear.

mismatch-repair gene: One of a set of genes whose function is to repair minor damage to the DNA molecule. Certain individuals have mutations in mismatch-repair genes. Minor degrees of DNA damage accumulate with repeated cell divisions and eventually cancer follows. Mutated mismatch-repair genes are found most commonly in patients with *hereditary nonpolyposis colon cancer* (q.v.).

mitochondria: Tiny cytoplasmic *organelles* (q.v.) responsible for the generation of energy (required for the cell's chemical reactions). Mitochondria also contain a tiny amount of DNA, acquired from the individual's mother.

mitosis: The process by which a cell splits and divides into two other cells. Each of the new cells has the same genetic material as the original cell.

mole: See *nevus*.

monoclonal: Arising from one cell. All cells in the monoclonal group or tumor show similar characteristics to the cell from which they arose. Cf. *polyclonal*.

monocyte: A type of white blood cell that can transform into a macrophage and ingest foreign debris or microbes.

mortality rate: Number of deaths from disease during a specific time (usually one year), divided by the number of people at risk.

MRI scan: Magnetic resonance imaging scan. An MRI scan builds up signals from the natural magnetic properties of cells and tissues to form a very precise anatomical picture of organs and tissues. In some circumstances it provides far more information than CT scans. In other circumstances CT scans are more appropriate.

mRNA (messenger RNA): A molecule that carries signals from the DNA in the nucleus to the ribosomes within the cytoplasm. In the ribosomes the signals are translated into amino acids and proteins.

MSH2 gene: One of the genes responsible for repairing minor DNA damage. It is one of the *mismatch-repair genes* (q.v.).

MTS1 gene: One of the *mismatch-repair genes* (q.v.).

mucosa: The delicate epithelial membrane that lines the inside of the mouth, intestinal tract, respiratory tract, and urinary tract. It also lines the inner aspect of most ducts.

multiple myeloma: A type of cancer derived from plasma cells (which originate from B-lymphocytes). Multiple myeloma arises in the bone marrow and, although usually slow-growing, it can rarely be cured.

mutation: Any structural alteration of a gene that results in the wrong message being sent to the cytoplasm causing a defective protein or function. Mutations can be acquired or inherited. Common inherited disorders are sickle-cell anemia, cystic fibrosis, and muscular dystrophy.

myeloblast: Primitive immature granulocytes. Acute leukemia arising from granulocytes is referred to as (acute) myeloblastic leukemia.

myeloid: Cells of the neutrophil or granulocytic series. Leukemias arising from these cells are called myeloid leukemia. The terms *acute myeloid leukemia* and *acute myeloblastic leukemia* and *acute granulocytic leukemia* are interchangeable. The terms *chronic myeloid leukemia* and *chronic granulocytic leukemia* are also interchangeable.

myeloma: See *multiple myeloma*.

myocytes: Muscle cells.

myosin: A protein present in abundance in muscle cells. It is the mai protein responsible for muscle contraction.

NCI: National Cancer Institutes. NCI is a subdivision of the National Institute of Health (NIH) and is responsible for most U.S.-government-sponsored cancer research funding.

neoplasm: Another name for a tumor. Although commonly used as a synonym for cancer, it also includes *benign neoplasms* (q.v.).

nephroblastoma (or Wilms' tumor): A childhood cancer that arises from primitive embryonic tissue in the kidney. See also *Wilms' tumor.*

neuroblastoma: A malignant tumor arising from the primitive neurons in the medulla of the adrenal gland.

neuroendocrine cell: A cell that shows some features common to endocrine and neural cells. Cancers arising from neuroendocrine cells often secrete hormones.

neuron: The motor and sensory cells of the central nervous system (brain and spinal cord). Neurons are the cells responsible for all forms of movement and for all forms of sensation. Someone with paraplegia or someone who has suffered a stroke loses function primarily from loss of neuronal activity. Tumors arising from the neurons are relatively rare; the commonest is the medulloblastoma arising in the brain (usually of children).

neutrophil: The commonest white blood cells circulating in the blood. They are also called granulocytes, polymorphonuclear leukocytes, and PMNs. They are the first protective cells to move to any site of tissue injury or infection. They are the main cells responsible for the acute inflammatory reaction.

neutrophil transfusion: See *granulocyte.*

nevus: A benign mole due to an accumulation of benign pigment-producing cells (melanocytes) in the skin.

NIH: National Institute of Health.

NM23: A gene whose function is not fully understood. It may play a role in preventing metastases.

N-myc gene: An oncogene that is commonly amplified in neuroblastomas (childhood cancer of the adrenal gland). When it is elevated neuroblastomas behave more aggressively. The presence of amplified N-myc worsens the prognosis.

nodes: Short for lymph nodes or lymph glands.

Non-Hodgkin's lymphoma: Malignant tumor of the T or B immune cells (lymphocytes), which arises most frequently in lymph nodes, but may arise in lymphoid tissue anywhere. It strikes middle-aged and older adults mostly. However, no age group is immune. Approximately 85 percent of all lymphomas are of this variety and they have various histological grades. Low grade tumors may need no therapy, whereas high grade tumors need aggressive chemotherapy, similar to that for acute leukemia.

norepinephrine: Also called noradrenaline, and like adrenaline a hormone that contributes to the speed and strength of the heartbeat and to the blood pressure control. See *catecholamines* and *epinephrine* for fuller discussions.

normoblast: The precursor cell of the red blood cell. Normally it is present only in the bone marrow. Under certain conditions it spills into the peripheral blood. An exceptionally rare form of leukemia arises from normoblasts and is called erythroleukemia or diGuglielmo's disease.

nuclear atypia: The dysplastic abnormal nuclei seen in cancer and premalignancy. Sometimes benign conditions can cause atypical nuclei and mimic dysplastic changes.

nucleus: The membrane-bound structure in the center of the cell. The nucleus consists of proteins and water and contains the cell's chromosomes and their genes.

occupational cancers: Cancers that have been associated with specific occupations such as shipbuilding (asbestos-related mesothelioma), uranium mining, dye manufacture, and the manufacture of polyvinylchloride.

oncogene: Genes present in normal cells that contribute to the regulation of cell growth. In cancer they may be amplified or overactive and drive the tumor cell to proliferate rapidly and out of control.

oncologist: Medically qualified doctor who specializes in treating cancer patients.

organ: Any fully formed tissue in the body such as heart, lung, brain, or kidney.

organelle: Tiny structures within the cytoplasm of the cell. Each type of organelle has a specific function. Examples of organelles are *lysosomes* (q.v.), *mitochondria*, (q.v.), and *ribosomes* (q.v.).

osteoporosis: The commonest form of bone disease. Pathologically osteoporosis is characterized by an absolute loss of bone tissue, especially in the spine. It is common in the elderly, and affects, in particular, postmenopausal women. It causes pain and fractures. Some forms of osteoporosis are secondary to other medical conditions such as *Cushing's syndrome* (q.v.).

osteosarcoma: A highly malignant tumor arising from bone-forming cells. It usually affects children and young adults. It can affect any bone. Most commonly it grows close to the knee joint.

p-arm: The short (petite) arm of a chromosome.

palliative treatment: Treatment aimed at alleviating pain and ensuring that the patient can live in relative comfort. It does not attempt to eradicate cancer completely.

pap smear test: The microscopic examination of cells taken from the surface of the cervix is named after Dr. Papanicolaou, who first used cytology for diagnosing cancer and precancer.

paraneoplastic syndrome: Symptoms that cannot be due to the size or anatomic location of the tumor. There are many types of paraneoplastic syndromes. Some are related to hormone-like substances secreted by the tumor, others are due to immunological reactions against normal tissue. Examples include muscle wasting, skin pigmentation, general physical wasting, and *Cushing's syndrome* (q.v.).

pathologist: A medically qualified doctor who specializes in the examination of tissue, blood, fluid, or secretions for diagnostic purposes. The term is most commonly used to describe surgical histopathologists who examine biopsied tissue microscopically. They diagnose, grade, and stage cancer.

PCR (polymerase chain reaction): A molecular biology technique for amplifying tiny fragments of DNA or RNA. After amplification the DNA or RNA can be analyzed.

peptide: A group of amino acids linked together. Amino acids and peptides are assembled to form proteins.

peripheral blood: Circulating blood in veins and arteries. The term peripheral blood cells is used to distinguish cells that are circulating in the blood from those that remain localized or fixed in the bone marrow.

peristalsis: Rhythmic contraction of smooth muscle in the intestine and some other tissues (such as ureters and bile ducts). The process of peristalsis helps to propel food forward and onward from the esophagus to the anus.

permanent cells: The small number of cells in the body that do not proliferate after birth. Examples of permanent cells are neurons and muscle cells in the heart. Cf. *labile cells*, *stable cells.*

p53 oncogene: The oncogene responsible for controlling many aspects of the cell cycle that also contributes to the control of apoptosis. It is mutated in more than 50 percent of all cancers.

pharmacologist: Scientist who studies the mechanisms and effects of chemical compounds (drugs).

pheochromocytoma: A tumor arising from adrenal medulla cells. Pheochromocytomas are usually benign but have profound hormonal and biochemical effects resulting from an elevated production of *epinephrine* and *norepinephrine* (q.v.).

Philadelphia chromosome: A translocation between chromosome 9 and 22 that is characteristically found in *chronic myeloid leukemia* (q.v.). Two oncogenes, *abl* and *bcr,* are juxtaposed at the translocation site and are thought to contribute to the development of leukemia.

physiotherapist: Someone who is trained to treat, advise, or assist in treatment by using physical exercise or massage.

pituitary gland: A pea-sized gland at the base of the brain that secretes a variety of hormones. Pituitary hormones control the activity of the thyroid, the adrenal glands, the ovaries, the testes, and body growth.

plasma cells: Cells present in the bone marrow and lymph nodes that are responsible for the manufacture of immunoglobulins and antibodies. Plasma cells are derived from B-lymphocytes. Malignancy arising from the plasma cells is called multiple myeloma.

platelets: Tiny cells that circulate in the peripheral blood and prevent bleeding by plugging damaged or cut blood vessels. They release numerous chemicals that contribute to blood clotting. Their deficiency, such as occurs in leukemia and lymphoma or after chemotherapy, may lead to widespread bleeding. Platelets are derived from megakaryocytes in the bone marrow.

ploidy: The total amount of chromosomal DNA in nuclei. The normal amount is referred to as euploid. Nuclei with abnormal amounts of DNA and chromosomes are said to be aneuploidy. Aneuploidy is common in malignancy and often correlates with the degree of biological aggressiveness.

PMNs: See *neutrophil.*

polyclonal: Having proliferated from different cells. Benign tumors are due to growth of cells derived from many different cells. In contrast, most cancers arise from the continued growth of a single cell. Cf. *monoclonal.*

Polymerase Chain Reaction: See *PCR.*

polymorphonuclear leukocytes (PMNs): See *neutrophil.*

polypectomy: Removal of a polyp by cutting or cauterizing its base.

polyps: Small protruding nodules derived from epithelial tissue. Sometimes the nodules are composed of benign tumor cells; these are benign neoplasms. Colonic polyps are typical examples. Approximately 1 percent become malignant. Some polyps arise from inflamed tissue and are not neoplasms.

poorly differentiated: Bearing little resemblance to the original tissue from which a tumor arose. In general, poorly differentiated tumors are aggressive. See also *differentiation.*

precancer: Cellular changes that precede cancer. A typical example is dysplasia of the cervical epithelium. Sometimes dysplastic changes revert to normal. Sometimes they progress to invasive cancer.

premalignant: Conditions that may progress to cancer over a long time, such as chronic ulcers, Barrett's esophagus, or colonic polyps.

primary tumor: The first or original tumor. The term is used to distinguish the primary tumor from metastatic tumors, which are sometimes referred to as secondaries. Theoretically, each organ in the body can be the site of either primary or secondary (metastatic) tumors. Occasionally the distinction between primary tumor and metastatic tumor may be difficult (for example, in the ovary). A patient may have more than one primary tumor.

prognosis: The long-term outlook for a patient with disease. For cancer patients it is commonly measured in terms of *five-year survival rate* (q.v.).

promoter: A chemical that completes the generation of cancer in a process of carcinogenesis started by another. The concept is theoretical, and in clinical practice it is not known how often the concept is recapitulated. What is clear is that carcinogenic agents frequently assist each other, in which case they are referred to as cofactors. For example, asbestos causes malignant mesothelioma (a malignancy of the lining of the lung) and cigarette smoking causes lung cancer arising from the bronchi. Cigarette smokers who are also exposed to asbestos have a much greater risk for developing primary lung cancer than those exposed to cigarette smoke only.

promoter gene: A gene that influences or controls another gene. Promoter genes play an important role in switching on or switching off those genes responsible for cell proliferation.

prostate specific antigen (PSA): An antigen that is secreted from prostatic epithelial cells. It is secreted in excessive amounts from prostatic cancer and is detectable in the blood, where its level correlates to some extent with tumor bulk. Doctors use the PSA test to screen for prostatic cancer or to monitor patients for tumor recurrence.

prosthesis: An artificial replacement of tissue or organ. Common examples are heart valves and hip replacements.

protease: An enzyme responsible for breaking down structural proteins. Tumors secrete proteases, which allow the tumor cells to invade and metastasize.

q-arm: The long arm of a chromosome.

radiation therapy: A form of cancer treatment in which radiation is directed at a tumor. Radiation may be used alone or in combination with surgery and chemotherapy. Some tumors are very radiosensitive, and in certain circumstances radiation therapy can achieve the same result as surgery. However, like surgery, it is confined to localized treatment of the primary tumor and its immediately adjacent tissues. It may also be helpful as a palliative procedure for reducing tumor bulk or pain—for example, with metastases to the spine.

radical lymph node dissection: Complete removal of an entire group of lymph nodes. Some cancers spread to draining lymph nodes and remain there for a long time before metastasizing widely. Under such circumstances radical removal of an entire group of lymph nodes may be curative. A common example is cancer of the larynx (voice box) that has spread to the lymph nodes in the neck. Radical dissection of the lymph nodes in the neck may prevent subsequent spread. The same principle applies to colon cancer.

radiobiology: The study of how cells and tissue respond to various doses and methods of radiation delivery.

radioresistant: Of tumors, unresponsive to radiation therapy.

radiosensitive: Of tissues or tumors, vulnerable to killing by radiation.

radiotherapist: A medically qualified doctor who treats patients with radiation therapy.

radiotherapy: See *radiation therapy*.

red blood cells: See *erythrocytes*.

retinoblastoma: A malignant tumor arising from the retinal cells in the eye. Sometimes retinoblastomas are hereditary and due to a mutation in the retinoblastoma tumor suppressor gene.

retrovirus: An RNA virus that uses the enzyme reverse transcriptase to convert RNA to DNA, which then integrates into the DNA of the host nucleus. It disrupts the normal coding sequence of the host DNA. The AIDS virus is a retrovirus. One particular form of T-cell leukemia common in Japan and the Caribbean region is caused by the retrovirus known as HTLV1 (Human T-Cell Lymphotrophic Virus).

Rhabdomyosarcoma: A malignant tumor arising from skeletal muscle cells anywhere in the body. This is one of the commoner malignancies in children. Most forms respond well to chemotherapy and are cured. In adults, they are rare, respond less well to chemotherapy, and generally have a poor prognosis.

ribosome: An *organelle* (q.v.) in the

cytoplasm of each cell that is responsible for converting the message from DNA into amino acids and proteins. Cells that manufacture abundant protein are particularly rich in ribosomes.

risk ratio: A term used by epidemiologists to quantify the risk of disease associated with a particular occupation or event or drug or any other variable. The measurement is made in comparison to what would happen if the variable was absent.

RNA: Ribonucleic acid. During the course of protein synthesis an instruction is transferred from the DNA in the nucleus to the ribosomes in the cytoplasm through a messenger molecule made from RNA. This is called messenger RNA or mRNA. There are other forms of RNA also present in the cell.

RNA virus: A virus whose core is made of RNA. Such viruses require the presence of the enzyme reverse transcriptase to change their RNA to DNA. This allows the virus to integrate into the host nucleus.

S phase: The phase during the cell cycle in which DNA is synthesized from existing DNA.

salivary glands: Small (a few millimeters) and medium-sized (a few centimeters) glands located around and outside the mouth that secrete fluid and digestive enzymes into the mouth (saliva).

sarcoma: A malignant tissue arising from connective tissue and mesenchymal cells. Sarcomas can arise from any tissue in the body. In general, they tend to be more malignant and less sensitive to chemotherapy and radiation therapy than carcinomas. However, their degree of malignancy is highly variable, and some forms are very sensitive to therapy (as, in particular, are many childhood sarcomas).

scar tissue: Connective tissue that accumulates at the site of previous tissue damage. Occasionally scar tissue continues to grow and can be confused with a tumor. For example, such scars on a mammogram may resemble a small carcinoma.

sclerosis: Dense connective tissue resembling scar tissue. It is benign.

screening cytology: Microscopic examination of cells in an attempt to detect premalignant changes. Screening cytology is carried out particularly in the prevention of cervical cancer. Cervical cytology, in which the doctor randomly removes cells from the surface of the cervix, is typical of screening cytology. Cf. *diagnostic cytology.*

SEER: The surveillance, epidemiology, and end results program of the National Cancer Institute (NCI) in Washington. SEER is one of the organizations that provides population-based cancer statistics in the United States.

segmentectomy: Surgical removal of a breast segment.

seminoma: A malignant tumor of the testes arising from germ cells. Seminoma is highly sensitive to chemotherapy and radiotherapy, and patients with this tumor have an excellent chance of complete cure. The same tumor occurs in the ovary, where it is called a dysgerminoma. It too arises from germ cells and has an excellent prognosis.

serosa: A membranous lining on the outer surface of almost all abdominal organs.

sigmoidoscopy: Endoscopic examination of the distal part of the colon (the sigmoid colon).

skin cancer: Any of three common skin cancers: *squamous cell carcinoma* (q.v.), *basal cell carcinoma* (q.v.) and *malignant melanoma* (q.v.). Only the last commonly metastasizes. The other two are slow-growing tumors readily treated by surgical excision.

smooth muscle: Muscle cells present in the walls of all contractile organs and tissues except the heart. Examples are the intestine, the uterus, and the walls of blood vessels. Benign tumors arising from smooth muscle cells are termed leiomyomas. Their malignant counterparts are leiomyosarcomas.

sporadic: Of cancer, occurring randomly with no hereditary background.

squamous cell carcinoma: A slow-growing skin cancer that rarely metastasizes. In this they are like basal cell carcinomas (q.v.). Squamous cell carcinomas in other organs are aggressive and metastasise.

stable cells: Cells that grow and proliferate when injured or stimulated. Normally they proliferate at a very slow rate and divide once every few months or possibly once a year. Liver cells behave like this. However, when a portion of a liver is removed, liver cells grow and proliferate rapidly to replace lost cells. Cf. *labile cells*, *permanent cells*.

stage: See *tumor stage*.

stem cells: These reside in low numbers in the bone marrow and give rise to all other marrow and blood cells. They can be induced by GCSF (q.v.), to proliferate and spill into the blood in large numbers where they are collected and returned later to the patient as a stem cell transfusion. Stem cells are collected when the patient is in remission for later use, if he or she should relapse. Stem cell transfusion has replaced bone marrow transfusion in most situations where a "marrow" transfusion is required.

stroma: See *connective tissue*.

suicide genes: A popular term for those genes controlling the process of apoptosis (q.v.).

T-cell leukemia: Leukemia derived from T lymphocytes. T-cell leukemias arise in adults and children.

TAF: See *angiogenesis growth factor*.

tamoxifen: An antihormone drug used in the treatment of breast cancer (mainly). It is particularly useful for tumors that are rich in estrogen receptors. Estrogens often enhance breast-cancer growth and in order to do this they must bind to estrogen receptors present in breast-cancer cells. Tamoxifen blocks the binding of estrogen to its receptor and thus removes the estrogen growth effect.

telomerase: An enzyme that maintains telomere length. Cancer cells have active telomerase that contributes to tumor cell immortality.

telomere: Segments of chromosomal ends that act as molecular clocks. Each time a cell divides it loses pieces of its telomeres. At some critical level of shortening, normal cells can no longer divide. Cancer cells have long telomeres due to the activity of *telomerase* (q.v.).

teratogenesis: The process by which radiation, chemicals, drugs, or other agents cause defects in the developing embryo.

teratoma: A type of tumor that recapitulates many of the tissues in a developing embryo or fetus. Skin, bone, brain tissue, and intestine may all be present. There are benign and malignant variants. About 10 percent of all ovarian tumors are benign cystic teratomas, also called dermoid cysts. Malignant teratomas can be found at any location but are commonly situated in the testes.

testosterone: Male hormone produced primarily by cells in the testes. Sometimes this hormone exerts a growth influence on prostate cancer.

thymine: One of the DNA bases that form the genetic code.

thymus gland: A small gland located behind the breast bone (the sternum) that is very important for the development of the immune system in the fetus and young child.

thyroid gland: A gland in the front of the neck, overlying the larynx (voice box), that is responsible for much of the body's metabolic activity. Radiation from the Chernobyl disaster caused a large number of thyroid cancers, as did radiation therapy in the 1950s for trivial conditions.

tissue: A general term used for layers of cells in any organ in the body. Each organ in the body is made up of thousands of cells that are bound together into layers of tissue.

transitional epithelium: The epithelial lining of the urinary bladder, ureters, and part of the kidneys.

translocation: Breakage at one part of a chromosome and relocation to another chromosome. Commonly the break results in loss of biochemical activity. However, in some circumstances the translocated genes interact with genes present at the new site to cause some new adverse effect, such as uncontrolled cell proliferation.

tubular adenoma: An intestinal polyp composed of glands. It is a benign neoplasm that rarely becomes malignant.

tubulovillous adenoma: A benign neoplasm of the intestine that has a similar low tendency as tubular adenoma to become malignant.

tumor angiogenesis growth factor (TAF): See *angiogenesis growth factor.*

tumor necrosis factor (TNF): A chemical that is released from immune cells in an attempt to destroy tumors. It has many activities; one of its most visible activities is cachexia (wasting) in cancer and AIDs patients.

tumor stage: The extent to which a tumor has spread from its original site. Many staging systems are in use; however, they are all based on similar principles. For convenience we can think of tumor spread as having three major steps. Stage I is when the tumor is confined to the tissue from which it has arisen. Stage II refers to tumor that has spread to draining lymph nodes. Stage III refers to tumor that has spread to distal organs such as liver or bone marrow. Often those stages have subdivisions, or frequently a four-stage system rather than a three-stage system is used.

tumor suppressor gene: A gene whose function is to slow down a particular activity, such as cell growth.

tumor type: The histopathologic classification, e.g., squamous cell carcinoma, adenocarcinoma, melanoma, lymphoma.

tumorigenesis: A general term used to describe the development and progression of cancer.

ulcerative colitis: A common chronic inflammatory disease of the colon. Its cause is unknown. A small percentage of patients with longstanding ulcerative colitis are at risk for the development of colon cancer.

ultrasound examination: An imaging technique using ultrasound waves to outline the size, shape, and consistency of internal organs. Its most common use is in assessing the development of a fetus *in utero*. However, many abdominal organs can be visualized very well using ultrasound. Its main advantages are that it is non-invasive and does not use any ionizing radiation (X-rays). It is very reliable in distinguishing cystic from solid tumors or tumorlike masses.

undifferentiated: In a tumor, one that shows no resemblance to the tissue from which it has arisen. It is a stage beyond *poorly differentiated* (q.v.). Most undifferentiated malignant tumors, no matter where they have arisen, tend to resemble each other, microscopically. See also *differentiation.*

urologist: A medically qualified doctor trained in the diseases and surgery of the urinary tract and male genital system.

villous adenoma: A benign polypoid tumor of the intestinal tract, usually the colon or rectum. Villous adenomas have greater malignant potential than tubular or tubulovillous adenomas, which are also polyps of the intestine.

Von-Recklinhausen's disease: A hereditary disorder characterized by the presence of benign neural tumors in the skin and elsewhere. Rarely these may undergo malignant transformation. The resulting cancer is a neurofibrosarcoma, also called a neurogenic sarcoma or a malignant schwannoma.

well-differentiated: Having a microscopic appearance very similar to normal tissue. See also *differentiation.*

Wilms' tumor (or nephroblastoma): A form of kidney cancer in infants and children. Most are sporadic. However, a small percentage is hereditary. Wilms' tumor and neuroblastoma are the commonest abdominal cancers in children.

WT1 gene: Mutations in this gene play a significant role in the development of Wilms' tumor.

Index

Numbers in **boldface** indicate illustrations (figures). A number followed by "(t)" indicates that the reference appears within a table on that page.

abl 103, 173
achalasia (esophagus) 58, 173
acquired immune deficiency syndrome (AIDS) 17, 48, 114
ACTH (adrenocorticotrophic hormone) 47, 173
actin 21
adenine 93, 173
adenocarcinoma **24**, 39, 173
adenoma 39, 61, 173
adhesion molecules 32, 97, 173
adrenal adenoma 39
adrenal gland 47, 81, 87, 88, 173
adrenaline 88, 173
advances in treatment 159
aflatoxin 109, 109(t), 110, 115
AGCT 93, 173
alchemy theory 12
aldosterone 88, 173
allele 173
allogenic transplant 138, 174
alternative medicine 139
amino acid 97, 174
androgen 56, 174
anemia 59, 60, 62, 69, 84, 97, 174
aneuploidy 89
angioneogenesis 34, 35, 101, 161, 164, 174
aniline dye 111
animal cancer 14, 115
antibodies 17, 36, 48, 69, 88, 161, 174
anticancer vaccines 115, 161
antigen 174
APC gene 118, 118(t)
apoptosis 19, 34, 36, 67, 68, 101, 174
Aristotle 11
asbestos 107, 109, 109(t), 111, 113
ascites 174
astrocytes 174
astrocytoma 85, 174
ataxia 174
ataxia-telangectasia 84
atrophy 27, 174
autologous bone marrow transplantation 137, 174
axilla 12, 43, 54, 124, 126, 131, 132, 174

B-cell leukemia 175
B symptoms 176
Barrett's esophagus 58, 124, 148, 175
basal cell carcinoma 112(t), 113, 123, 132, 157, 175
base 93, 97, 103, 175
basement membrane 30, **31**, **32**, 33, 50, 98, 123, 175
basophils 175
BcL2 oncogene 19, 175
bcr oncogene 103, 173
Beckwith-Wiedemann syndrome 82, 87, 175; *see also* Wilms' tumor
benign prostatic hyperplasia 175
benign tumors (neoplasms) 24, 39, 42, 50, 74, 116, 119, 123, 124, 148, 175
biopsy 176
Bittner agent 14
black bile theory 11
bladder cancer 44, 72, 108, 109(t), 110, 111, 116, 117, 156
blast transformation 67, 69, 176
blood, normal cells 83
Bloom's syndrome 84, 176
bone marrow 83, 176
bone marrow transplantation (BMT) 137, 176

brachytherapy 133, 176
brain tumors 40(t), 85
BRCA1 118(t), 119, 148, 176
BRCA2 118(t), 119, 148, 176
breast cancer 11, 12, 14, 34, 36, 39, 40(t), 43, 49–54, 150; hereditary factors in 118(t), 119, 148
breast lumps, benign 50
bronchoscopy 47, 49, 176
Burkitt's lymphoma 113, 114(t), 176
busulphan 111

CA-125 71, 156, 176
cachexia 176
carcinogen 106–119, 177
carcinoma in situ **31**, 51, 54, 60, 73, 98, 122, 150, 151, 152, 177
carcinosarcoma 177
case control studies 107, 177
castration 177
catecholamines 88, 177
CD34 138, 177
CD44 35
CDK Inhibitors (CDKI) 101
cell 15, **16**, 177
cell cycle **25**, 26, 177
cell membrane (cell wall) 16, 32, 36, 135, 138
centromere 177
cervix, cancer of 32, 75(t), 114(t), 116, 122, 123, 124, 129, 152, 156, 162
chemical carcinogenesis 110
chemoprevention 161
chemotherapy 6, 17, 19, 23, 25, 44, 49, 54, 56, 65, 68, 71, 73, 74, 85, 86, 88, 89, 101, 110, 111, 112(t), 129, 132, 133, 135, 177
Chernobyl disaster 83, 112
childhood cancer 81–90
chondrosarcoma 42, 177
chromosomes 20, 37, 61, 69, 87, 91, **92**, 99, 103, 118, 157, 178
cigarette smoking 110, 117, 124
cilia 178
cirrhosis of the liver 115, 178
clinical trials 36, 64, 89, 107, 136, 142, 161, 162, 178
CLL (chronic lymphocytic leukemia) 67, 178
clone 30, 35, 98, 101, 129
clustering of cancers 82, 178
CML (Chronic Myeloid Leukemia) 67–69, 103, 178
cohort study 107, 178
colectomy 179
colon cancer 39, 60–64, 101, 111, 116, 117, 118(t), 124, 131, 148, 160
colonoscopy 63, 149, 179
colostomy 179
columnar cells 179
complementary medicine 139
computer language 94, 95, 115
conformal radiotherapy 134
congenital cancers 81
connective tissue 18, 34, 42, 45, 49, 87, 89, 123, 179
cortisol 179
craniopharyngiomas 86, 179
Crick, Francis 93
CT (computerized tomography) scan 43, 49, 65, 122, 128, 179
Curie, Marie 112
Cushing's syndrome 39, 47, 179
cyclin-dependent kinases (CDK) 101
cyclins 101
cyst 179
cystic fibrosis 99, 148, 163
cystoscope 73, 179
cytochemical profile 179
cytogenetics 93, 103, 179
cytokines 17, 179
cytologist 179
cytology 179
cytoplasm 15, **16**, 36, 48, 95, 97, 114, 135, 180
cytosine 93, 180

DCIS (ductal carcinoma in situ) 51, **52**, 98, 123
Denys-Drash syndrome 87
deoxyribose 180
dermis 180
desmosomes 32, 180
diagnostic procedures 48, 55, 121, 127, 180
diethylstilbestrol 180
differentiation 15, **18**, 34, 39, 40, 40(t), 42, 46, 56, 101, 110
differentiation genes 20, 48
DNA 15 26, 30, 54, 61, 74, 81, 89, 93, 114, 118, 119, 129, 133, 135, 148, 150, 154, 156, 180
DNA virus 181 *see also* viruses
Down's syndrome 84
Duchenne's muscular dystrophy 163
ductal carcinoma (breast) *see* breast cancer

ductal carcinoma in situ *see* DCIS
Dukes staging 63, 181
dysphagia 181
dysplasia 14, 30, 45, 55, 58, 62, 98, 116, 123, 124, 129, 145, 156

Ebers papyrus 11
economics of cancer care 9, 155, 159
ectoderm 18, 181
Egyptians 11
electromagnetic fields 82, 113
electron microscope 14, 15, 19, 32, 47
embryo 13, 181
embryonal theory 13
emphysema 181
endoderm 17, 181
endometrium 110, 126, 181
endoplasmic reticulum 16, 181
endoscope 55, 58, 73, 124, 181
enzymes 15, 17, 26, 34, 45, 57, 97, 98, 99, 114, 135, 181
eosinophil 181
epidemiology 6, 9, 59, 81, 107, 116, 145, 156, 159, 160, 164, 182
epinephrine (adrenaline) 88, 182
epithelium 182
Epstein-Barr virus 113, 114(t), 181
erythrocyte 182
esophageal cancer 58, 109(t), 117, 156
estrogen and progesterone receptors 54
European Commission's International Agency for Research on Cancer 7
Ewing's sarcoma 89
exons 93, 182

false negative diagnosis 182
familial adenomatosis polyposis (FAP) 61, 117, 118, 118(t), 124, 148, 183
Fanconi's anemia 84, 183
fetus 183
FHIT gene 183
Fibriger, Johannes 14
fibroadenoma 50, 126, 183
fibrocystic change 183
fibroid 183
fibrous tissue 183
fine needle aspiration cytology (FNAC) 183
five-year survival rate 183
fragile sites 183
French-America-British (FAB) classification 84, 182
future developments and trends 159

G phases 26
G zero phase 26
Galen 11
gastric cancer 14, **59**, 66, 109, 109(t), 111, 125, 131, 157
gastrointestinal cancer 57 *see also* gastric cancer
gastroscope 183
GCSF 183
gene rearrangements 129
gene therapy 20, 103, 162, 183
genes 15, 19, 21, 25, 30, 31, 34, 36, 48, 61, 67, 74, 81, 87, 89, 91, 118, 118(t), 119, 129, 148, 160, 162
germ cell cancers 72
glandular mucosa 184
Gleason grading system 56, 184
Glioma 40(t), 184
grade 184 *see also* tumor grade
granulocyte colony stimulating factor (GCSF) 6, 184
granulocytes 67, 68, 83, 184
guanine 93, 184

Harvey, William 12
Helicobacter pylori 184
helix 184
hematologist 184
hematoxylin 184
hemoglobin 184
hemophilia 163
hemoptysis 184
hepatitis B virus (HBV) 114(t), 115
hepatocellular carcinoma 115
hepatocytes 26
hereditary cancers 117, 118(t)
hereditary nonpolyposis colon cancer (HNPCC) 61, 118, 118(t), 184
Hildanus 12
Hippocrates 11
Hiroshima and Nagasaki 112
history of cancer 11
Hodgkin's disease 65, 85, 133, 185
homeobox genes 20, 185
hormone 185
HOX genes 20
HTLV1 (human T-cell lymphotrophic viruses) 82, 84, 114, 114(t)
Human Genome Project 103
human papilloma virus (HPV) 114(t), 116, 124, 154, 162, 185
hyperplasia 27, 28, **28**, 55, 129, 185

hypertrophy 27, 28, **28**, 185
hysterectomy 185

immune cells 17, 26, 40(t), 42, 60, 65, 137, 185
immunoglobulins 69, 185
immunotherapy 185
infectious mononucleosis 114
infectious theory 13
information, obtaining 141
inhibitor genes 163
initiation 110
Internet 142
introns 93, 185
ionizing radiation 112, 133

junk DNA 93, 103, 185

KAI1 gene 37
Kaposi's sarcoma 114, 115, 185
karyotype 91, 185
keratinocytes 17
kidney, cancer of (renal cell carcinoma) 20, 74–75, 81, 87, 118(t), 156

labile cells 26, 27, 186
Laetrile 139
laparotomy 128, 186
larynx (voice box), cancer of 75(t), 109(t), 117, 155
Le Drun, Henry François 12
Leeuwenhoek, Anton van 12
leiomyoma 186
leiomyosarcoma 40(t), 42
leukemia 5, 29, 40(t), 42, 67–69, 81, 83, 85, 89, 109(t), 112, 112(t), 114, 114(t), 115, 137, 145, 166, 186
Lewis, Ed 20
Li-Fraumeni syndrome 101, 118(t), 119, 186
limb-sparing surgery 6, 132, 186
liposarcoma 40(t)
lobular carcinoma 51, 52
lobular carcinoma in situ (LCIS) 52
local spread (invasion) 186
lumpectomy 51, 123, 186
lung cancer 39, 5, 20, 40(t), 44–49, 81, 101, 111, 113, 117, 109, 109(t), 125, 150, 155, 160, 164
lymph nodes 12, 17, 24, 34, 35, 40(t), 43, 44, 46, 51, 54, 56, 63, 65, 67, 68, 73, 127, 131, 132, 134, 186
lymph theory 12
lymphatics 12, 15, 17, 25, 34, 35, 123, 186
lymphedema 132
lymphoblast 186
lymphoblastic leukemias 67, 83
lymphocytes 17, 26, 35, 40(t), 60, 64, 65, 67, 69, 83, 84, 114, 138, 186
lymphoma 5, 40, 40(t), 42, 60, 64, 81, 85, 113, 114, 114(t), 129, 133, 186, 187
Lynch syndrome 118

M phase **25**, 26, 188
macrophages 17, 186
magnetic resonance imaging (MRI) 36, 86, 122, 128, 152, 188
Malpighi, Marcello 13
mammography 9, 33, 51, 54, 122, 123, 129, 146, 147, 150, 187
mastectomy 187
Medline 143, 187
megakaryocytes 83, 187
meiosis 187
melanin 187
melanocytes 23, 187
melanoma, malignant 23–25, **24**, 40, 75(t), 112(t), 113, 123, 132, 147, 157, 162, 164, 187
meningioma 86
mesenchyme 187
mesoderm 17, 187
mesothelioma 109, 113
messenger ribonucleic acid (mRNA) 95, 97, 161, 187
metaplasia 27, 45, 58
metastases 29, 30, 34, 34, 43, 44, 47, 49, 51, 54, 56, 63, 71, 73, 88, 89, 98, 123, 127, 132, 134, 155, 157, 160, 162, 164, 187
micrometastases 187
microscope 12, 30, 34, 43, 44, 47, 49, 51, 54, 56, 63, 73, 71, 88, 89, 98, 123, 127, 132, 134, 155, 157, 160, 162, 164
mismatch-repair genes 99, 118, 187
mitochondria **16**, 17, 187
mitosis **25**, 26, 41, 54, **92**, 96, 188
MLH1 61, 118(t)
mole, pigmented **24**, 123, 124, 188
molecular biology 14, 15, 54, 67, 103, 116, 124, 129, 148, 154, 161
monoclonal proliferation 129, 188
monocytes 17, 188
Morgagni, Giovanni Battista 12
mortality rate 188
MRI scan *see* magnetic resonance imaging
mRNA *see* messenger ribonucleic acid
MSH2 gene 61, 118(t), 188

MTS1 gene 36, 188
mucosa 188
Müller 13
multidrug resistance 130, 135
mutations 30, 61, 70, 74, 95, 98, 99, 101, 113, 118, 118(t), 119, 129, 148, 150, 156, 188
myeloblast 188
myeloid 188
myeloma (multiple myeloma) 69, 188
myocytes (muscle cells) 21, 27, 40
myosin 21, 188

Napthylamine 109, 109(t)
National Cancer Institute (NCI) 5, 6, 142, 144, 188
National Center for Health Statistics 6
National Library of Congress 143
neoplasms 39, 188 *see also* benign tumors
nephroblastoma 188 *see also* Wilms' tumor
neural network (artificial intelligence) 129, 154
neuroblastoma 88, 100, 188
neuroendocrine cell 188
neuroma 86
neuron 189
neutrophil transfusion 189
neutrophils 17, 83, 189
nevus 24, 189
nipple discharge 50
nitrosamines 58, 59, 110, 109, 109(t)
Nixon, Richard M. 5
NM23 Gene 36, 189
N-myc gene 89, 100
no threshold hypothesis 112
non-ionizing electromagnetic fields 82, 113
norepinephrine (noradrenaline) 88, 189
normoblasts 83, 189
nuclear atypia 189
nucleus 15, 20, 21, 30, 36, 91, 94, 95, 97, 115, 119, 189

occupational cancers 189
oncogenes 54, 89, 99, 101, 103, 189
oral cavity and pharynx, cancer of 75(t)
organelles 15, 189
osteoporosis 189
osteosarcoma (osteogenic sarcoma) 40(t), 42, 89, 189
ovary, cancer of 70, 110, 137, 156

p-arm (of chromosome) 190
P21 gene 101
P53 oncogene 36, 101, 118(t), 119, 130, 164

Paget's disease of the nipple 50
palliative treatment 190
pancreas, cancer of 40(t), 46, 75(t), 107, 156
Pap smear test 9, 32, 152, 154, 190
papillary carcinoma 40(t)
papillomaviruses 114(t), 154, 162
Paracelsus 20
paraneoplastic syndromes 47, 88, 125, 190
parasitic theory 13
pathologists 31, 36, 42, 49, 52, 65, 66, 87, 121, 124, 126, 129, 132, 153, 154, 159, 190
peptide 190
peripheral blood 190
peristalsis 190
permanent cells 28, 190
pharmacologist 190
pheochromocytoma 190
Philadelphia chromosome 69, 103, 190
pituitary gland 190
plasma cells 190
platelets 21, 83, 84, 138, 191
ploidy 191
polyclonal 191
polycyclic hydrocarbons table 109(t), 110
polymerase chain reaction (PCR) 129, 154, 190
Polymorphonuclear leukocytes 17
polyps, colon 61, 117, 124, 148, 149, 191
Pott, Percivall 106
preinvasive cancer 31, 123, 150, 151
primary tumor 191
progesterone receptors 54
prognosis 191
promoter 191
promoter genes 21, 163, 191
prostate cancer 5, 8, 37, 39, 54–57, 101, 119, 122, 127, 134, 146, 154, 160
prostate specific antigen (PSA) 55, 127, 155, 191
prosthesis 191
protease 192

q-arm (of chromosome) 192

radiation therapy 33, 49, 51, 54, 56, 65, 74, 86, 89, 101, 112, 112(t), 123, 127, 133, 192
radical lymph node dissection 192
radioactive iodine (I^{131}) 134
radioactive isotopes 133, 161
radiobiology 134, 192
radioresistance 192
radiosensitizers 162

radon 113
rectal cancer *see* colon cancer
red blood cells 13, 21, 83, 84, 97, 138, 182
retinoblastoma 81, 89, 118(t), 119, 192
retroviruses 14, 84, 114, 192
reverse transcriptase 114
rhabdomyosarcoma 42
ribonucleic acid (RNA) 95, 97, 114, 192
ribosomes 15, **16**, 48, 95, 97, 192
risk ratio 192
RNA *see* ribonucleic acid
RNA virus 192 *see also* viruses
Rokitansky, Karl von 13
rous sarcoma 14

S phase **25**, 26, 192
saccharin 108
salivary gland 192
sarcoma 193
scar tissue 193
Scheurlen 14
Schistosoma 116
sclerosis 193
screening for cancer 9, 32, 54, 55, 62, 87, 89, 121, 122, 129, 145
SEER 6
segmentectomy 193
seminoma 193
serosa 193
sickle-cell anemia 98
sigmoidoscopy 149, 193
skin cancer 193 *see also* melanoma, malignant
small intestine, cancer of 60
Smith papyrus 11
smooth muscle 193
sporadic cancers 193
squamous cell carcinoma 40, 40(t), **41**, 45, 58, 112(t), 123, 193
stable cells 26, 27, 193
staging cancer 12, 42, 49, 54, 56, 59, 63, 65, 73, 71, 74, 87, 131, 133, 136, 149, 189,
statistics 6, 7(t), **8**, 75, 75(t)
stem cell transplantation 85, 137
stomach cancer *see* gastric cancer
stress, cellular response to 23
suicide genes 193 *see also* apoptosis

T-cell leukemia 193
TAF *see* tumor angiogenesis factor
Tamoxifen 54, 193
telomerase 99, 161, 194
telomere 194
teratogenesis 194
teratoma 194
testis, cancer of 2, 75(t), 134, 156
Thiersch 13
Thorotrast 112, 112(t)
thymine 93, 194
thyroid, cancer of 40(t), 75(t), 83, 112, 131, 133, 136
thyroid gland 194
tissue 10, 194; organization and differentiation 15
transitional epithelium 194
translocation 194
traumatic origin theory 13
treatment 4, 5, 9, 42, 84, 131, 143, 162
tubular adenomas 62, 194
tubulovillous adenomas 62, 192
tumor angiogenesis factor (TAF) 35, 174
tumor classification 39, 40(t)
tumor dormancy 36, 82, 135
tumor grade 41, 42, **43**, 132, 133, 184
tumor necrosis factor (TNF) 35, 194
tumor staging 194
tumor suppressor genes 87, 99, 100, 119, 194
tumor terminology 39
tumor type 195
tumorigenesis 195

ulcerative colitis 61, 124, 148, 195
ultrasound examination 70, 74, 87, 137, 155, 156, 195
ultraviolet (UV) radiation 111
undifferentiated cancer **41**, 195
urologist 195
uterus, cancer of 40(t), 42, 75(t), 126

vaccines for cancer 115, 161
vagina, adenocarcinoma of 82
Vesalius, Andreas 12
VHL gene 74
villous adenomas 62, 195
vinyl chloride 109(t), 110
Virchow, Rudolf 13
viruses 14, 84, 113, 114, 114(t), 115, 124, 154, 162
Von Hippel-Lindau syndrome 74, 118(t)
Von Recklinhausen's disease 118(t), 119, 195

Watson, James Dewey 93
Wilms' tumor 74, 81, 87, 118(t), 195
World Wide Web (WWW) 4, 142, 144
Wt1 gene (Wilms' Tumor Gene-1) 87, 195